INTERPERSONAL RELATIONS

AND

THE EROTIC EXPERIENCE

DR. JORGE WEIBEL SAEZ

Dedication

A posthumous tribute to my parents, simple folks with a great vision of the importance of educating their children.

IV

Acknowledgments

I gratefully acknowledge the collaboration and patience of Diane Garzón, María Zajia and Claudia Figueroa, who were instrumental in improving the manuscript more than once.

A special thanks to the Costa Rican writer Dr. Rima Vallbuona for her interest and effort in going over the manuscript. I am indebted to her for her contribution to making the book easier to follow.

I thank Dr. Eleodoro Peña Ramos for his recommendations that made the text more accessible to young readers, and Dr. Carlos Martínez for furnishing bibliographic material that was crucial for the completion of some chapters.

Dr. Erik Weibel helped with the design and review of the book to make it more attractive. Without his help during a particularly rough period of my life this book would not have been possible. I am deeply grateful.

I thank Michelle Francesconi for her help with proofreading this book.

I appreciate the work by Victor Almansar for his excellent illustrations which complement the understanding of the text.

I also thank Dr. Heles Contreras for his invaluable help in the translation of this text from Spanish to English.

I am also indebted to my immediate family, who through a retrospective analysis of our years together allowed me to value the importance of a satisfactory interpersonal relation for the harmonious coexistence of couples and the individual development of children. Unfortunately there was a void in many aspects of family life, due to lack of knowledge and experience and also to working conditions, which did not make it possible to devote more time and attention to the needs of every family member.

I also thank Rose Gloor, Mariana Staforelli, and Fernando Staforelli for their help in the design of the cover of this book.

Finally, I thank all the people that allowed me to interview them. Their personal experiences contributed important material to the book.

Table of Contents

DEDICATION III

ACKNOWLEDGMENTS V

PROLOGUE X

INTERPERSONAL RELATIONSHIPS 14

    Attraction...16
    Communication 18
    Acceptance 19
    Sharing...20
    Purpose 20
    Appreciation 21
    Relationship development 23
    The loving relationship..24
    Deterioration of the relationship...................................24
    Romantic illusions and fantasies 27
    "We are in love" 29
    True or false love 31
    Passionate excitement..35
    Infatuation..37
    Love and sex 39

LOVE...44

    Definition...44
    Scientific research 44
    Socio-cultural evolution 45
    Biological considerations 46
    Anatomical basis of love 49

Emotional instability 50
Explosive laughter and crying...50
Aggressiveness, violence, anger, rage, and fury....................51
Indifference and apathy 52
Alterations of sexuality..52
Socio-cultural aspects..53

THE EROTIC EXPERIENCE..59

FOREPLAY 62

ANATOMY OF THE SEXUAL ORGANS.......................................63

The male genitalia 63
Corpora cavernosa of the penis 71
Female genitalia..72
The ovaries 72
The uterine (or Fallopian) tubes 73
The uterus 74
The vagina 76
The anatomic basis of the sexual act/neurophysiology 79

SEX HORMONES..83

Testosterone..84
Estrogen..86
Progesterone 87
Prolactin..87

PHYSIOLOGY OF INTERCOURSE 89

The male sexual act 89
Phases of the male sexual act 90
Erection...90
Lubrication 91
Emission and ejaculation..92
The female sexual act 93
Phases of the female sexual act 94
Stimulation 94

Erection and lubrication 95
Orgasm...95
Resolution or relaxation phase 99

VAGINAL PENETRATION POSITIONS 100

ORGASM 106
Determining factors 106

KEGEL'S VAGINAL EXERCISES 118
Directions for vaginal exercises 119

ORAL SEX 120

ANAL SEX 125

PREMATURE EJACULATION...127
Treatment...129

DELAYED EJACULATION 134

MASTURBATION 136

STRESS REDUCTION 140
The fight or flight response 142
Methods of relaxation..145
First Phase 148
Second Phase 148
Third Phase..149
Personal experience 151
Concentration and attention..151
Calm, serenity, self-control, peacefulness 152

ABOUT THE AUTHOR..154

REFERENCES 156

Prologue

The publication of a new book on human sexuality, about which so much has been written, calls for justification. The idea of writing this book goes back over more than fifty years when I started my professional practice. That it has taken a few years to write it is due to the fact that the scientific information required appeared periodically over a long stretch, as we will see below, and the acquisition of clinical data has required an extended period of clinical practice. Furthermore, the acceptance of public discussion of human sexuality has taken a few decades. For this reason, medical consultation relating to sexual problems was limited. Male patients would discuss primarily their inability to get an erection or the problem of premature ejaculation. Female patients would normally talk about their inability to obtain sexual pleasure, so-called anorgasmia.

The problem that we doctors faced was the lack of adequate training for the treatment of these difficulties. Medical schools did not offer courses on human sexuality. The neurophysiology of the sexual organs and the sexual act was not well understood. The first studies on these matters appeared only in the late sixties. Neither was there an understanding of the psychological factors that would make it possible for an interpersonal relation to ensure a harmonic and lasting co-existence. A satisfactory erotic experience, especially for women, depends greatly on the existence of a harmonious relation. This is also important in the relationship between the couple and their children during their psychological development.

The first studies on human sexuality were published in the forties by Dr. Alfred Kinsey. He showed that only 30 per cent of married women were able to get an orgasm. Another important piece of data in these studies was the high percentage of divorces (about 50 per cent), which holds true even today.

There was also a high percentage of sexual impotence among males older than 50, and premature ejaculation among younger males. Another important fact was the high number of unplanned pregnancies among single women under 20, about one million per year. Concerning the latter problem we must keep in mind the hormonal activity that occurs at this stage. Most young men are sexually active, but not so many young women are. The erotic feeling aroused by petting may lead to sexual intercourse. A young woman may resist, but the fear of abandonment may force her to go along. The young man will see the woman's surrender as proof of love, but very often he does abandon her after she gets pregnant. Young couples think that their affection for each other makes it socially acceptable to engage in sexual activity that may ruin their lives in exchange for 20 seconds of pleasure.

To avoid the problems associated with pregnancy young couples are increasingly engaging in oral sex. The use of condoms has caused much controversy, since some people think it facilitates promiscuity. The tendency among conservatives is to recommend abstinence before marriage. Abstinence is an excellent preventive measure, but it is very hard to practice. With due respect to political and religious considerations, abortion makes sense in certain special cases, like incest, rape, or when the mother's life is at risk or the fetus shows abnormalities that would prevent a normal development. For married couples that have all the children they want, there are safe medical procedures that prevent pregnancy, like tying the male's spermatic cords or the female's uterine tubes. Women should have control over their bodies and be free to undergo or reject abortion.

During the sixties William H. Masters and Virginia E. Johnson published their work concerning the favorable results obtained by applying psychotherapy to sexual problems. Unfortunately their results were not duplicated by other scientists. Around the same time and in the early seventies, there appeared the first studies on the neurophysiology of the sexual organs, in particular the ones involved in the sexual act between a man and a woman. These findings made it possible to use medicines in the treatment of sexual impotence and premature ejaculation.

In the Latin culture there are fathers who encourage their sons to have early sexual relations with a woman provided by them, usually a prostitute, to make "men" out of them. Some mothers get their gynecologist to prescribe contraceptives for their 16-year old daughters to prevent any problems. This can have serious consequences, since the pill contains a hormone that produces thrombosis in the arteries of the brain, causing cerebral infarction. Traditional moral principles require women to practice chastity and remain virgins until matrimony. But times have changed, and not all young women follow this path. Instead they let themselves be influenced by television, movies, and novels, with their veiled suggestion of sexual activity.

In spite of the importance of sexual education for young people, there is much controversy surrounding it, since there is no agreement on how, when and where it should take place and who should do it. The main problem is not the difficulty of providing the relevant information, but the discussion of sexuality itself. This should deal with the sexual function of both sexes, including the anatomy and physiology of the genital organs, their biological function, the expressions of sexuality during the individual's development and maturation such as masturbation, the nature of erotic pleasure and its function in interpersonal relations, how to satisfy your partner sexually so as to develop a lasting and harmonious relationship, how to facilitate an interpersonal relation, how to avoid the risk of failure and the negative effect of inexperience, and how to avoid unplanned pregnancies and sexually transmitted diseases like AIDS.

Parents find it very difficult to have open discussions of sex with their children but they can provide useful and simple advice as to how to avoid unplanned pregnancies and sexually transmitted diseases. Parental attitudes are probably due to lack of knowledge about human sexuality or the fact they have been in the same situation as their children. Parents should understand that the purpose of sexual relations among young people is to get erotic pleasure. For married couples, 99% of sexual relations have the same purpose. Procreation accounts only for 1 %.

There are some erroneous views concerning how a man can satisfy his wife. There is a TV ad about a product that can cure erectile dysfunction where the woman attests to the efficacy of the product by asserting that after months of unhappiness, depression, and the sense that their married life makes no sense, she has now regained her happiness since her husband can achieve a stronger and more lasting erection. This ad suggests that a stronger and lasting erection is sufficient for a woman's sexual satisfaction. This is false. There are husbands, including physicians, who after a few years of not practicing foreplay, believe that having an erection is a sufficient stimulus for their partner to be sexually aroused, and practically force her to have sex. This behavior on the part of the husband is misguided, and the sexual act becomes traumatic and humiliating for the woman. It is in fact a form of rape. Understandably, many of these relationships end up in divorce. There are also many wives that "have sex", as opposed to "making love", only to satisfy their husbands.

This book offers information on these mistaken ideas and on the sexual practices that should be avoided in order to achieve a stable, lasting, and mutually satisfying interpersonal relation.

The book is intended for parents, physicians, medical students, nurses, social workers, and psychologists. Here they will find useful information that will improve their professional practice.

Interpersonal Relationships

Interpersonal relationships start at birth. By biological necessity, the newly born establishes a relation with his or her mother, who is responsible for providing food, nourishment, and care. The baby's mother provides love and establishes a harmonious bond to ensure that the baby develops in a secure and loving environment.

Fathers must also establish an early personal relationship with newborns, by holding them and helping to bathe them and change their diapers whenever possible. This relationship must continue until the child reaches independence.

The infant learns to recognize emotions and affection not only by being fed and cared for. Human skin is the body's largest organ that keeps us in contact with the environment. The receptive cells located in the subcutaneous tissue are the means of communication with everything that surrounds us. There are specialized mechanisms to register temperature, pain, and touch.

Touch is perhaps the most important means of registering the parents' affection until the development of language and the ability to distinguish between pleasant and unpleasant things. The expression of affection through touch is appreciated not only by infants but throughout the entire course of life. A pat in the back, a handshake, a hug, a caress on the face are signs of love and affection that everybody appreciates.

Expressing emotions in this way is important for the establishment and development of an interpersonal relationship. It is particularly desirable for parents to engage in these practices with their children as they grow up.

Grown-ups should know and keep in mind that many parts of the skin are sensitive to touch and caressing. For women the most sensitive areas are the neck, behind the ears, the nipples, the groin, the interior part of the thighs, the abdominal surface, the clitoris and the vagina, more specifically the vaginal labia.

These areas are for the most part erogenous. Their stimulation facilitates the sensual arousal prior to lovemaking. A woman once stated on TV that all she required to get aroused was for her nipples to be caressed.

There are also erogenous zones for men but they are less sensitive than those for women. Manual or oral stimulation of the penis is the major source of arousal leading to erection and orgasm.

Interpersonal relationships provide the most meaningful opportunities for emotional development and maturity in the course of our existence. Each relationship reveals something about us. We seem to attract people who one way or another awaken in us certain aspects of our inner selves and our environment. They allow us to discover what goes on inside ourselves and to clarify our negative attitudes, thoughts and feelings. There is in each of us a certain type of energy or dynamism that constitutes an important part of how we interpret what happens in our lives. This is why it is important to reflect daily on our attitudes to make sure that they are correct and that we maintain a clear vision of our feelings. If we are not aware of what we feel or what is happening within ourselves, we are unable to make decisions or react to other people in such a way as to make justice to our true feelings. We may then experience highs and lows in our interpersonal relationships and end up with adverse effects in our day-to-day existence. Interpersonal relationships must involve respect, consideration, appreciation, and emotional satisfaction for everyone that we come in contact with.

In this chapter I will highlight interpersonal relations in the development of emotional growth mainly in the context of love and the erotic relation between couples.

I will also try to provide a basis on which parents can establish a close connection with the members of their immediate family. The family environment should be a source of learning to foster a positive interaction with children, something that is too often neglected, with negative repercussions for children after they leave home.

A thorough appreciation of the erotic and loving experience begins with the understanding of the dynamic governing interpersonal relations. The affective or erotic communication of a couple will certainly reflect the emotional state of the moment. Worries, frustrations, and mental anxiety resulting from adverse home experiences will necessarily affect a person's ability to give or receive love openly and thoroughly. We must do our best to fully understand our interpersonal situations so as to be able to change any negative aspect that might interfere with our ability to love.

It is necessary to consider the different phases that might facilitate mutual understanding. In our every day existence, as well as in clinical practice, it is clear that our interpersonal relations are often unsatisfactory. This is true not only of romantic relations but also of family life, the work place, and any other activity that calls for a harmonious relationship in order to achieve a more positive outcome.

Keeping in mind the importance of the interpersonal dynamic in the romantic and erotic experience, we will describe certain phases of the process that will contribute to achieve better mutual understanding. This will not only help us get a better sense of the romantic and erotic relation but will also be useful for other activities where mutual relations are important.

ATTRACTION

Attraction is likely to be the first factor triggering the onset of an interpersonal relation. There are different types of unilateral or mutual attraction. For men in particular, attraction towards the opposite sex comes mainly from visual perception. Women are aware of this fact, and respond to it by the care they take in personal appearance.

For women, physical attraction is not as important as respect, attentiveness, and good manners. Attraction may be reinforced by the existence of common interests in social, artistic, intellectual, or sport activities, among others. The ease with which attraction may lead to the establishment of a relationship depends on the ability or desire to reach mutual communication. In cases where attraction is based on one factor alone and is limited by an intellectual differential, both the initial relationship and its future development will have a weak foundation. If, on the other hand, the relationship is reinforced by involvement in common activities, its prospects for success increase.

Knowledge of each other starts with the first encounter of a couple. The main factor that triggers the relationship is attraction. It is ideal for this attraction to be mutual, but in some cases there is unilateral attraction, and the person who feels it tries to maintain an attitude that will earn him or her the attention of the other party. Mutual attraction must not be confused with what is called "love at first sight", since in this first encounter there is nothing more than the spontaneity of interest or attention, and the couple may not be aware of what their emotional and affective reactions are.

Interpersonal attraction is highly variable. This attraction, as we have said, may result from visual perception. If this is the case, the attraction in question is physical. The physical characteristics that are considered appealing vary from one person to another. This is to be expected, since mass media highlights certain physical characteristics of men and women as representative of a visual standard of "beauty". When there is no exposure to mass media, it is early experiences that determine which physical qualities are appealing. Thus some people may be attracted by specific parts of the body. Others may be attracted by general physical appearance, demeanor, attitude, voice or manner of expression, attire, economic situation or profession. Women are more likely than men to use attire as a means of attraction. For men, who are generally more experienced than women in this area, the attraction is openly sexual. The first impression may be so intense that it determines future choices so that we always opt for somebody who resembles the person who made that first impression. Attraction may be initially superficial and grow stronger as we get better acquainted with our object of attraction. It is also common that the choice represents an act of rebellion against one's parents. It may also be the case, if the person has few chances to relate to the opposite sex, that the choice is made just because the opportunity presents itself. Whatever the case, attraction is always necessary as a starting point for the relationship.

COMMUNICATION

Communication is the key to success in any kind of relationship, be it in the work place, with our spouse, lover, parents, children or friends. It is essential to establish the means of communication that allow both parties to express their feelings and needs.

In particular there must be a method of communication that allows each party to express his or her desires without humiliating the other party and without a dominating attitude. To achieve this we must be willing to listen to the other person with respect and full attention so as to ensure that the message has been accurately transmitted. It may be that what is said and what is received do not match. True communication starts with total respect for the other person as a human being. If we are not willing to communicate our thoughts and feelings or if we are not receptive to what may hurt us and refuse to listen, the relationship has little chance to develop.

Communication is essential for the establishment of an interpersonal relationship. We know that not everybody has the same ability to communicate. Communication must be spontaneous, open, sincere and honest. Both parties must express their feelings and desires clearly. The meaning of the transmitted message must be apprehended by the hearer without distortions or misunderstanding. The person transmitting the message must make sure that the meaning intended was accurately conveyed. Communication makes it possible to reveal what we are and to project through dialogue our wishes, opinions, judgment and cultural level. The art of communication goes beyond just the simple transmission of information; it may also serve as an expression of love.

This is important when a woman receives a message from a man. If our mode of expression is not honest and sincere, we will project a false image of ourselves that will eventually be revealed as such. It is very hard to maintain an unnatural and false façade. Sooner or later the mask will fall and our deceit will be revealed.

One aspect of communication between a man and a woman involves the recognition of their differences. This acknowledgment is unfortunately very rare in practice, a fact that contributes substantially to the problems that couples experience. We differ in how we feel, think, express ourselves, interpret things, and how we give and receive. Failure to acknowledge these differences may lead to a deterioration of a relationship. When a woman discusses her problems she does it primarily to express her feelings and to satisfy her emotional needs. She wants not only to communicate with the other person but also to be heard. If she is listened to with empathy, she feels validated, understood and supported. When a woman talks about her problems she is not looking for solutions. It is important for men to learn how to listen. This is an art that can be learned through practice. The man must learn how to interpret what the woman wishes to communicate. The woman may repeat herself in order to grab the man's attention and feel that her emotional needs are met.

Men need a reason to talk. They do not speak just to share something. They do it to look for solutions to their problems; because of this they erroneously tend to propose solutions when a woman talks about her emotional needs.

But men also want their emotional needs to be satisfied. If a man feels accepted, trusted, appreciated, admired, it will be easier for him to listen to his partner and offer her the understanding that she needs and deserves. Consequently if both the man and the woman feel that their basic emotional needs are satisfied communication becomes easier and more satisfying. The main problem for the modern couple is not money, as frequently thought; it is communication.

ACCEPTANCE

Another essential element is acceptance. We must learn to accept each other with dignity. Acceptance of another person does not imply that we share all their ideas and actions. At the beginning of an interpersonal relationship we must be willing to accept the other person as he or she is, just as we would want to be accepted. This acceptance must be unconditional, open, and spontaneous. We must shed our self-defense mechanisms as we engage in the process of acceptance. It is important to generate or feel empathy so as to facilitate the initial interaction and allow us to act more freely as individuals. Otherwise, if acceptance is conditional, tension will arise and the genuine expression of appreciation will be made more difficult.

It is crucial to show respect for the other person's beliefs, political ideas, good or bad qualities, personal characteristics, viewpoints or opinions on any areas of their interest. It is not fair to try to change them, since we also want to be accepted as we are. It is important to learn to respect differences and thus feel closer to other people.

SHARING

We all have our own personal preferences and inclinations, but there may also be common interests and activities that can be pursued together. We must respect individual preferences and not try to impose our own desires. Sharing contributes to a sense of unity, support, and partnership. It might be desirable to engage in alternating or reciprocal participation in an activity that appeals to one of the parties as a show of solidarity. This might reinforce the sense of unity by showing support for your partner. It also acknowledges the sense of personal independence, a necessary condition for the pursuit of individual interests such as music, painting, sports, hobbies, etc. Joint participation in the erotic experience is sharing each other's sensual pleasures.

PURPOSE

Once communication has been established we must ask ourselves: What is my purpose in this relationship? What do I want to do? What is the intended course of this relationship for me or the other person? Is this a short-term or a permanent relationship? The relationship will not be well defined unless there is an understanding and sense of purpose for both parties. Otherwise we will be operating on false premises. Each party needs to define his or her situation, rules of conduct, and boundaries. If the parties differ and one person is willing to contribute more than the other, the relationship will be on shaky ground. Each person must concern himself or herself with the well being of the other as much as his or her own and commit himself or herself to solving problems together and maintaining the lines of communication open.

Clarifying the purpose of the relationship is of paramount importance since it guarantees that both parties will know in advance what the boundaries are and the frustration or pain of an unexpected breakup is avoided. The duration of an interpersonal relationship can only be decided on after a reasonable period of getting to know each other. This mutual knowledge is possible only if both parties participate in open and honest communication concerning the purpose of the relationship.

APPRECIATION

An often forgotten factor is appreciation. We do not tolerate situations where we feel unappreciated. If we think of any relationship that makes us unhappy, we will see that one way or another what is at the bottom of it is a lack of appreciation. If we do not show appreciation for what others do, if we fail to make others feel special, we generate negativity and insecurity. A pat in the back or a kind word is an easy sign of appreciation, but we seldom take the time to offer it. An attitude of appreciation signifies that one is sensitive to the needs of others. We should keep in mind that a woman's self-image and self-esteem are threatened when her partner fails to pay attention to her. Showing appreciation for a person signifies that he or she is special. Little things that may not mean much to a man may be very important to a woman. When a man ignores something that is valuable to the woman, she feels ignored. If men knew what these "little things" mean to women there would be many more happy women. A little note, a card, a phone call can be signs of love that make a woman feel special and give her the sense that her emotional needs are being met. Women need tokens of love. A bouquet of flowers, for instance, may convey not only that her partner loves her but may also reaffirm her beauty and femininity.

Men generally assume that once a woman is satisfied she will continue to be. Once he has shown his love, she should not need reassuring. This sounds logical to a man. Women, however, find this attitude difficult to accept. It is totally inconsistent with their internal reality. They need to be reassured that they are special, and that they are loved and appreciated.

Men also need reassurance. They feel stimulated when they are needed and appreciated for their ability to succeed and get results.

Women need above all to be supported. They feel stimulated and secure when they are appreciated and respected. A sympathetic attitude validates the significance of any statement, feeling or situation.

A respectful attitude conveys to the other person that their rights, wishes and needs are important. By showing respect we communicate that we value the other person as he or she is and that their needs matter to us. This is the kind of attitude that makes us truly be at the service of the other person because he or she deserves it.

An attitude of appreciation acknowledges the value of the other person's effort and behavior and leads naturally to the sense of feeling protected. The attitude of acceptance signals to the other person that his or her behavior has been well received. It is also accompanied by a sense of gratitude for what we have been given. The attitude of trust is an indication that the other person's positive attributes – honesty, integrity, truthfulness, sincerity, sense of justice – are recognized and appreciated.

Appreciation of others is encapsulated in the Christian humanitarian precept "Love thy neighbor as thyself". It is not easy to love oneself, since it requires knowledge of what we really are. Many people believe they love themselves when they really do not know who they are. Love of oneself is important because without it we are likely to be insecure and afraid and to misinterpret the actions and words of those around us. In order to begin loving ourselves we must learn what is good and what is bad in us. If we concentrate on what displeases us in our environment we emphasize the negative. If, on the other hand, we focus more on our positive attributes we counteract what we don't like.

Acknowledgment of our flaws is an expression of honesty that others appreciate, but it is more important to correct them and to concentrate on our positive traits. It is common for a woman to feel that she is no longer loved because her partner has stopped giving her the same attention that he gave her at the beginning of the relationship. When the quality of attention changes, the woman – without a full understanding of how men are – concludes that he is unhappy and that she no longer matters to him. Attentiveness is the most important token of love.

RELATIONSHIP DEVELOPMENT

The factors discussed above contribute to the establishment of a mutually satisfying interpersonal relationship. We must keep in mind that the success of the relationship depends on the extent to which these factors exert a positive influence on the couple. It may be that not all these factors are present, but the more there are the better the chances for a positive and stable relationship. If, on other hand, the relationship is based on only one or two of these factors, chances are that it will be unstable and fragile. For instance, if the attraction is mainly sexual or based on the need to satisfy one particular need of one of the parties, it is quite possible that the relationship will deteriorate once the need in question has been satisfied. This is quite clear when the only interest is to attain a favorable economic situation, to have a child, or to escape a difficulty home situation. In such cases the relationship is based on a very limited and selfish motive that will not contribute to the development or even the possibility of the other factors we have discussed.

It is true that in some cases the relationship starts out on the basis of one or two factors but these are eventually complemented by others. It must be admitted, however, that this is not the most common situation. Teenagers and young adults lack the necessary knowledge that would allow them to enter into a harmonious and stable relationship to develop a satisfactory mature partnership. Our early experiences at home, the example of our parents, relatives and friends, what we read in magazines, what we see in movies or on television, all of this is psychologically disorienting. It does not add up to a consistent set of values.

We learn through the media that couples experience selfishness, disloyalty, deceit, envy, hatred, violence, uncontrolled ambition, and romantic fantasy. On the other hand, our social environment is very unstable, and does not favor the possibility of developing interpersonal relationships that can evolve throughout long periods of time. There are demands that take precedence, like getting a degree, getting a job, or starting a business. This makes it difficult to start a relationship.

In addition to the general lack of knowledge concerning the factors that contribute to the development of an interpersonal relationship, there may be difficult temporary situations that must be faced. If we add to this the existence of limited financial resources and of social, cultural and religious differences, the full development of a relationship becomes very difficult. It is, nevertheless, very important to focus on what really matters, so that the relationship is based on real human factors that lead to harmonious coexistence and not on romantic illusions or fantasies.

THE LOVING RELATIONSHIP

The purpose is to find the person with whom we can establish a stable affective relationship. Love is not something that can be found. What we need instead is to find the person with whom we want to establish this kind of relationship. Attraction by itself may be very superficial at the beginning. We must know if we are prepared to invest the time, energy, and dedication that are required by love. When we are ready to accept this responsibility, we are in a position to find somebody with whom to establish a relationship of mutual love. Love is an emotional attitude that connects and unites us with another person in a context of sharing. Mentally, love manifests itself as understanding. Emotionally, love is expressed through empathy. Physically, love is shown through touching and sexual fulfillment.

DETERIORATION OF THE RELATIONSHIP

Through the educational process we have been taught the basic tools that will allow us to develop our intellectual capacities and to acquire a profession to ensure our economic wellbeing. If we have the favorable material conditions that make this possible, the realization of our objectives will depend mainly on our interest, personal effort, perseverance, and dedication.

The instruction we receive at home is generally very incomplete in the social aspect. The cultural, religious, and sport activities that take place through school or home are limited and sporadic. Many people have no other social contacts than the personal interaction with coworkers, which eventually makes it hard to learn the basic principles of human coexistence. There are, to be sure, some opportunities to join groups of people with common interests, but they are limited. Besides, not all of these associations offer diverse opportunities for different age groups or people with different needs. It is important that young people have access to social activities so they can integrate themselves to their social environment and develop interpersonal relationships.

Attraction, communication, acceptance, purpose, and appreciation will help to establish an interpersonal relationship, which can develop into the deeper affective union we call love. If these factors foster the establishment of a spiritual and emotional union, why is it that relationships can deteriorate and sometimes end up in exactly the opposite behavior to what people want? We have often witnessed the breakup of a couple that for years gave the impression of being the 'ideal couple'. Why?

First of all, we must take into account that most people are not acquainted with the factors discussed above.

Second, relationships often start on the basis of a limited and superficial attraction that is assigned too much value.

Third, the relationship may not reach the level of communication required for the free and spontaneous exchange that makes it possible to express what bothers us or what we dislike about the relationship. Our fear to say what we feel prevents us from communicating what we ought to communicate. What are we afraid of? What is it that we do not want to communicate? These are questions that must be faced honestly if we want to keep the communication channels open. It may very well be that the main cause of breakups is lack of communication. Sometimes we are afraid to hurt the other person with what we need to say. But if we don't say what we need to say at the appropriate moment, the damage might be greater if the other party finds out about it by other means. If mutual trust gradually deteriorates, communication becomes more and more precarious.

Fourth, if acceptance of the other person has failed to develop in the course of time, the willingness to accept will diminish. If the cause of displeasure becomes evident and one of the parties changes their behavior or accentuates the defects, the attraction reaches a very low level and acceptance becomes impossible. Family problems, illness, financial, social or work conditions could induce tension that will cause a change in behavior. Coexistence then becomes unsatisfactory and can lead to intolerance.

Fifth, if the relationship was a short-term affair, it is bound to end once the need that motivated it is satisfied. If the terms of the relationship were clearly and precisely spelled out at the beginning, whatever the original purpose, ending it will satisfy both parties and there will be no emotional trauma. What matters is to know that the agreement was made honestly and with full awareness by each of the parties.

Problems arise when the terms of the relationship are ill defined or were not fully spelled out at the beginning. This may lead to the perception that the relationship lacks a purpose. There is no goal that can be visualized as years of living together. The accomplishments are sporadic and unimportant. The lack of direction may also have been caused by events and causes beyond the couple's control. Those who survive this absence of purpose may develop a conformist attitude. Let us keep in mind that in the course of time people's attitudes, interests, motivations and viewpoints change. It becomes harder to sustain an enthusiastic attitude. Thus, the combined effect of depression and resentment may foster the lack of appreciation for the importance of a sense of purpose.

This failure to develop a sense of purpose may also be due to health problems, family interference, financial difficulties, and environmental factors like new jobs and emotional insecurity.

When the situation is analyzed openly and realistically, we must appreciate the value of what has been accomplished, but we must also acknowledge that which was not achieved, be it for lack of foresight or knowledge of what the future offered, taking into account the many factors that contribute to the success or failure of our endeavors.

We can conclude that during our development, mainly as children and adolescents, we are not provided the necessary knowledge to establish interpersonal relationships based on solid foundations as opposed to appearances or romantic illusions. If we realize early on that the relationship we want is based essentially on our emotions, we must realize that these are ephemeral and make us incapable of recognizing our errors and use reasoning and logic. This does not mean that interpersonal relationships must be based entirely on logic, without an emotional component. There must be a balance between reason and emotion. This is what makes us human, perhaps divine, in the process of a loving relationship. A thorough understanding of the factors that make for a satisfactory and lasting interpersonal relationship is crucial.

It is not a simple and easy task. Even if we had a full curriculum including general knowledge in the humanities and the sciences and we added religion, good manners, sexuality, and above all the factors that make for a harmonious human relationship, there is no guarantee of success, mainly if education does not reach the masses and in general those who show no interest in knowing themselves and others better.

ROMANTIC ILLUSIONS AND FANTASIES

In this area we will consider what is probably the most common illusion, "love at first sight." This is no doubt one of the finest sensations. Our heart beats rapidly, we get goose bumps, our ears buzz, our whole body burns, and we feel like we are walking on air. There are few experiences in life that are so moving, overwhelming, and deceiving. What we normally call love at first sight is not really love. It may be little more than a strong and powerful attraction. We may be attracted to money, power, or curiosity as to what the other person represents. Many of these sources of initial attraction are included in the romantic formulas beautifully depicted in films. The playful verbal exchanges between the lovers are really a kind of dialogue that soon gets boring in real life. For instance, when a millionaire young man meets a poor girl in a movie, the story grabs our attention, since they have nothing in common outside of the screen. Lovers in movies always look attractive, thanks to makeup and the clothing that is available to them. In real life, anybody who believes that his or her partner will look as good in the morning as in the previous evening should not expect the relationship to last very long. Attraction at first sight, no matter how intense, is not a sufficient basis for a loving relationship. There is no great mystery or magic in "love at first sight". It is easy to get this kind of romance since its requirements are minimal: a little money, some attention, and sexual desire. If to this we add possessiveness, a bit of greed, and an attractive appearance, this kind of false love may be generated several times a day.

True love is something entirely different. Despite what all the romantic mythology says, true love is not instantaneous. One can find a partner any place, but we don't find love while walking on the beach, when we attend a party, or when we check people out in a bar. True love is not a feeling that captures us magically when a particular person enters our life. A true union based on genuine love is something that develops and solidifies in time when two people make a commitment to one another in mutual trust. In its initial period true love may manifest itself as a passionate feeling of "being in love", but this is not always the case. In other words, true love may or may not start as "love at first sight." The myth of "love at first sight" goes hand in hand with the myth that there is only one true love for each person.

We can say that in general we all start very early to develop an image of the person with whom we would like to have a loving relationship, start a family, etc. The source of this image is rooted in our exposure to fairy tales. Then as we grow up we are influenced by romance novels, and later the love stories that we see in movies make a big impact in our minds because of everything that surrounds the couple in love. The physical beauty of the stars, the dialogue and its intonation, all of this gives a model for how to act in order to woo the person we are interested in. On the other hand, we must not forget the influence of those around us during our growing years. Our father or our mother may awaken the image of what we want in our eventual partner. Also the attraction of the first people emotionally associated with our early experiences may become the pattern for the physical and psychological qualities of the person we seek. We must not forget also that these desirable qualities that may determine our choices come from our own being. There are those that openly state that whoever they marry should be well off, because they would like to have a comfortable existence. Others would like their future spouse to be attractive, affectionate, tolerant, etc. These requirements probably go back to early frustration and lack of affection during the development years.

The desire to find a person with the required attributes may be so strong that one can convince oneself that the person one finds actually has them even though this may not be the case. It is not unusual that a person who clings to a variety of requirements will fail to find the ideal person and go through unsatisfactory and short-lived relationships. This is why we stated above that it is important to keep in mind that we are not perfect. When we establish a relationship we must allow for a margin of tolerance and an understanding of acceptance of each other as we really are. We will thus avoid love fantasies.

"WE ARE IN LOVE"

"Being in love" may be one of the emotional stages of interpersonal relationships often manifested after a first encounter involving a strong mutual attraction. It may correspond to what is called "love at first sight." It may happen to some women deceived by the presence of a strong sexual attraction. They may think that because they have lain in the same bed and made love they "are in love." Just the fact that the sexual encounter was satisfying is not enough to assume that one "is in love." Most likely one "feels in love" due to a pleasant temporary sensation that makes one emotionally blind. This is nothing but another romantic fantasy or illusion generated by the satisfaction of a casual encounter.

To be in love is much more than a strong mutual attraction or the pleasant sensation that goes with sexual attraction and consummation.

Even though the true certainty of being in love arises out of an intense mutual attraction, it only becomes a reality when there is sharing of feelings, desires, motivations, similar interests, acceptance of individual differences, and a reciprocal appreciation that is difficult to define. As we see, this kind of attraction is not limited to just one aspect of a person; it involves the whole person in all its facets. It is global and mutual attraction. Its foundation is broader and more solid than an isolated, momentary, and superficial impression. Being in love implies spontaneous, broad, and uncompromising communication. The relationship becomes more intimate and stronger as the couple accepts each other as they are, respecting their differences and shortcomings. Their bonds are strengthened as they share responsibilities and enjoy either common or individual interests. Their emotional needs are satisfied as they receive the appreciation that they each require. The intensity of the affection may vary, but it does not disappear. The couple remains united in the fulfillment of the purpose of their union.

Being in love is an emotional process that develops gradually in the course of harmonious, respectful, loyal, and honest coexistence. It is more complicated than we imagine and very few people attain it. Erotic satisfaction is a consequence of the existence of this interpersonal affective relationship, not its cause.

It is more accurate to say that we "feel in love" when we are in an emotional state resulting from the intense attraction produced by a pleasant casual encounter. As an emotional state, this feeling is transitory and will disappear as soon as the attraction that originated it dies out. There are couples for whom the interpersonal relationship suddenly ends, after swearing they are in love. This is not the case when the relationship is anchored in the manner we have described, that is, when there is a true bond and people are genuinely in love. It is important to make a clear distinction between the true affection that lasts during a couple's coexistence and the romantic fantasy or illusion that lends a transitory basis to the interpersonal relationship.

We even hear on occasion children from four to eight years old saying that "they are in love." We could imagine that they are copying what they see on television or in magazines. In these cases there is no sexual intention. Kindergartens and coeducational schools may play an important role in the establishment of these relationships. I believe this is nothing but the need for companionship and the desire to play together and share activities. It is a friendly relationship.

When asked why they think they are in love, children will commonly say things like: "because I like him (her)", 'I like his/her face". Sometimes they just say "I feel that I love him (her)" without further explanations.

We should not concern ourselves unduly with this type of relationship, but children should be supervised when they are together. They should not be allowed to play unsupervised in a bedroom, since some seven- or eight-year olds are sexually precocious.

Most likely the relationship will end in time, since there will be other opportunities to establish relationships in the future.

TRUE OR FALSE LOVE

The word "love" may mean different things to different people, so it is hard to define it. One can say that love involves a special emotional state between two people, in particular between a man and a woman. Several psychological factors converge towards the harmonious development of a loving relationship. There are no rules or pattern to guarantee that a personal interaction will lead us to this affective state or condition. True love exists when nobody is trying to change anybody.

In interpersonal relationships we must carefully distinguish between "true love" and "false love." The latter has a way of inexplicably disappearing in a few weeks, even after what may have been considered the "romance of the century." This false love may be the first, the last, or any romantic involvement we have had. It if often exciting, sometimes fascinating, almost always seductive, because it is based on our favorite illusions. Unfortunately it is so seductive that it sabotages our chances to attain true love.

Unlike false love, true love involves not just an emotional relationship but also one of personal maturity. It acknowledges that feelings, like people, evolve in time and maintain intimacy through profound changes. True love is mutual, honest, and highly complex. People who truly love each other have enough faith in each other so they do not need extravagant presents or to faint in public. What matters is trust, respect, support, understanding, and the satisfaction of emotional needs. True love is the union of two people, not an exhibition or drama. It is a conscious choice, not a sensation or a magical state of being. It enriches your life and makes it more satisfying, but it is not a panacea that will solve all problems. Unfortunately, true love does not conquer all. Nobody can make the honeymoon last forever. One difference between true and false love is that the latter ends with the honeymoon. If the relationship continues it is only because the lovers try to recapture the initial passion. True love instead urges us to go forward without regretting the past. Flirting comes and goes, but trust becomes stronger and mutual interest increases. No wonder false love is frenetic and wild. It shines with romantic baubles. It makes attractive promises that true love never offers. Above all, it may reinforce the illusions about love acquired during childhood, starting with the myth of sleeping beauties and the images of television and movie stars and their engagements. On the other hand, our parents' and friends' relationships in real life may be imperfect and they may offer perplexing images of marital life that would normally be unacceptable to a young person's idea of a "perfect" love.

Most people spend a good part of their lives trying to reduce these contradictory impressions to something that looks and feels good, something that could be thought of as true love. Sometimes our feelings of love may be based on a pleasant sexual experience or excitement; sometimes they are based on beauty, power, wealth, social status, or security. Many of these romantic illusions are reflections of the false love we internalize during our youth.

False love is more common than we imagine. We often attribute to the person whose love we want attributes and feelings that do not exist in real life. We believe that we will find the perfect partner, that we will be intensely attracted to him or her, that we will rarely quarrel, that we will not want to be apart, that sex will always be satisfying, that we will never be sexually attracted to anyone else, that we will never need anybody else in our lives, that romance will last forever. These are some of the powerful illusions that make it difficult to imagine any other, more realistic, kind of love.

In our search for this impossible dream we have probably experienced a number of unsatisfactory encounters. Each one of them may satisfy our expectations for a while, but then they will vanish, leaving us confused, wondering why we failed and why we keep choosing those who in the long run are not the people that match our desires.

At the risk of sounding anti-romantic, we must say that true love has more to do with the mutual desire to share certain goals and commitments than with passion. This does not mean that passion is absent in true love, but its intensity and presence are not always constant or invariable. When passion diminishes, lovers continue to actively express affection, support, attention, and mutual tolerance. In genuine love there is balance between individual independence and mutual support and protection. Individual changes and development test the relationship but they do not threaten it. The absence of this balance is an indication that the relationship is too fragile. From the moment the parties in the couple feel and spontaneously express the desire to love each other and understand that this balance is an important ingredient of true love, they will accept this challenge. One of the signs of false love is that given any problem, it will withdraw, instead of facing it and looking for a solution.

We should each analyze our behavior in our past and present relationships. We should contemplate our feelings and focus on our actions towards our partner observing his or her reactions. What is the difference we are seeking between a loved one and a friend? What degree of commitment do we want? How willing are we to pursue it? How well do we know the other person? Are kisses and flowers the only tokens of love? Do we support each other as individuals beyond the relationship? Does our attitude show tolerance, respect, consideration, and support?

If we keep asking and answering these questions honestly, we will eventually begin to see some behavioral patterns that may help explain why true love escapes through our fingers. There are individuals who are attracted by people who want no commitment, perhaps because they themselves are afraid they lack the sincerity required by true love. This is obvious in cases where a person is chosen to impress one's friends and not because of any interest in him or her. Others, afraid to be left alone, take the first attractive offer that presents itself, which places them in an uncomfortable position with respect to each other and their friends.

If there is no true balance in sympathy, trust, intimacy, the desire to acknowledge an emotional need, the pleasure of sharing, giving and receiving, love does not exist. Similarly, if there is no interest in providing a sense of well being, in showing appreciation and attention by remembering an anniversary; if we do not take the time to share affection, mutual interests, to talk about what displeases us or about other problems that interfere with a harmonious relationship; if we are not willing to communicate, discuss differences and day-to-day situations in an open manner, but without hurting our partner; if we are not willing to do this, there is no love, and we have chosen the wrong person to establish a loving relationship.

If we concentrate and analyze the situation carefully so that we can identify the romantic illusions and fantasies that have ruled our past love life, it will not be difficult to determine if the present love is real or false. We should ask ourselves: What is different now? Is it the intensity of feeling, the quality of our sexual life or the fabulous time we had in our vacation? Do we accept each other as individuals as much as we adore each other as lovers? Can we listen to each other and answer our questions openly and honestly? Do we set aside our selfishness and personal pride and accept the challenge to work together for a better future? Honest answers are crucial in order to determine if our relationship is based on true love.

If a person wants to initiate a relationship, he or she must start by getting to know the other person and determining if he or she is potentially the right person, before speaking of love. We have said before that love cannot be found, only the person with whom we want to establish an affective relationship. This person can be anywhere, and nobody can tell us where and when we will find this compatible person that we can love.

We must stop thinking in superficial terms of attraction and ask above all whether one is prepared to invest the time, energy, and dedication that true love requires. Only when we accept this challenge will we be in a position to find someone that will return our love.

We must take into account that before opening our arms to anybody there are questions that need to be answered. We must evaluate any person we are interested in with respect to certain characteristics or traits matching a set of honest and realistic, not just apparent, priorities. This list will naturally reflect the values, beliefs, and personal goals of the person who is seeking a partner. Let us remember that in practice we must not be too strict with our criteria; otherwise it will be very difficult to find a suitable partner. Remember nobody is perfect. It is not wise, on the one hand, to try to establish a loving relationship with someone lacking the traits that we consider crucial. On the other hand, it makes no sense to create a fixed image of out "ideal partner." We must accept imperfections, make concessions and compromises, recognizing that this attitude is essential in the process of loving.

PASSIONATE EXCITEMENT

Passionate excitement is an emotional experience yet more intense than "love at first sight", but this does not make it more significant. It is characterized by the participation of both parties in the loving process and accompanied by an intense feeling of closeness, union, and ecstasy that is both wonderful and dangerous. When people are in this state they truly believe they are part of the other person, that they think alike and feel the same emotions. Literally speaking, one person fuses with the other, but this does not mean that they share the same experience. They can look at each other, caress each other and feel each other's heartbeats, but they cannot feel what is really happening inside each other. This means that there is deceit in excitement. They can both feel they are equally excited, only because their own desire is so powerful that cannot imagine anything different. Even when they both claim "to be in love", their separate perceptions may be very different: one can be excited about the relationship, the other about sex. When a person is in this state it is very difficult to overcome their own emotions to the point where they have a clear perception of what their partner really feels.

There is a tendency to believe that our partner is perfect because we tend to see only what pleases us the most. Passion blurs many of the emotional and mental defenses that normally warn us about the imperfections and shortcomings of the other person. Fantasies cover up all that is unknown in the situation. If one person tries to impress the other at the beginning, he or she will tend to show only his or her good points, which makes the relationship look marvelous. This helps intensify fantasy and create unrealistic expectations. This is no doubt the greatest danger of excitement and the first illusion to vanish.

So, all of a sudden, after a few weeks of ecstasy, we begin to notice that our partner's laughter is rather strident. He wants to watch football on TV, and she prefers to watch her favorite soap opera. The lovers start to think that they are no longer in love and to realize that they are not one and the same person. This discovery may in fact mark not the end but the beginning of true love, provided they are each willing to abandon the illusions they had about one another. Unfortunately, once we convince ourselves we are in love, it is easier to hang on to the illusion than to abandon it. We talk ourselves into believing that this emotional state will last forever and will erase all shortcomings. Passionate excitement makes us feel at least temporarily powerful and makes us blind to the world around us. When the couple is together it creates its own world: an oasis of satisfaction and happiness, disconnected from everything but its own pleasure. Passionate romance changes nothing in our lives. The greater our expectations of it, the greater our frustration when we return to reality. In fact, it is often the case that the more intense the passion the sooner the relationship ends. This is due in part to the fact that instant passion is based on superficial impressions that block the perception of serious conflict and differences. Once the relationship has failed, one can blame the other person for the breakup or conclude that the relationship was a mistake. In fact, the error is to believe that the feelings experienced in the state of excitement or passion will automatically lead to love.

There is nothing wrong with enjoying the state of excitement, provided one is aware that it will not last and keeps one's emotions in perspective. In fact, unless one confuses excitement with true love, the experience itself may be beneficial. In general, the only way one can analyze one's needs and preferences in love is through experience with other people. Very few people commit themselves to true love without having first known the other person for a reasonable period of time. Experience through time allows us to control our tendency to act under the influence of passion. It is dangerous to let oneself be guided by passion and it might lead to situations and behavior that will later be regretted. It is wise to anticipate every type of seduction in each new romantic relationship, and not lose sight of other priorities just because one feels attracted to another person.

In order to establish a secure interpersonal relationship, the couple must go beyond the passive illusion of falling in love and begin the process of loving each other. This entails accepting and understanding the imperfections, flaws, and problems of each other as well as learning what each one needs from the other. In true love, once the stage of excitement is over, there is no need to feel lost in the other person. Both people feel more secure and aware of themselves as individuals. This is not an overnight process but a gradual development through time. As the romantic relationship evolves the risk of excitement diminishes. It is thus possible to set aside superficial impressions and open the way to the development of a true interpersonal relationship.

INFATUATION

The interpersonal relationship in which feelings and affections arise in an obsessive, absorbent, and explosive manner leads to the state of infatuation. In certain respects, this resembles excitement, but the dynamics of the relationship are more intense and dominating. In this state, there is total submission of one to the other. In some cases, one plays the role of a slave unconditionally at the service of the other. The need for mutual affection or for dominance is such that it allows no independent behavior. Spontaneity, individual freedom, and independence are lost. Submission is practically total, as there is almost no chance to escape. Self-realization becomes difficult due to insecurity and fear of losing one's partner. This insecurity extends to the future, perceived as uncertain and offering no possibilities for self-realization. This is most commonly the case in relationships involving teenagers. The home situation is generally unsatisfactory. Parents, for one reason or another, are unable to offer their children affection, understanding, or to listen to their emotional needs. The feeling of loneliness and the need for affection are pressing. The psychological changes they undergo during puberty make them feel insecure, alone, and without support. The hormonal changes that happen at this age make them seek the company of the opposite sex, looking for romantic love more than sexual gratification. An 18 year old young woman put it this way: "My mother doesn't understand me; I love him, I want to be with him all the time, eat with him, live with him, sleep with him, without any sexual desire towards him. My mother doesn't understand that something like this can exist..."

On the other hand, parents may be too strict, without understanding that their children have a social need to interact with their peers. This creates a sense of mistrust on the part of the children.

The situation becomes critical if the young people are part of families that do not accept each other socially. In these cases, the relationship may proceed openly and defiantly, or in secret. Both situations create anxiety and insecurity. Isolation and the need for affection make the young people more dependent on one another.

The situation becomes catastrophic when the parents of one or the other disapprove of the relationship. Fantasy replaces reality, and clinging to their romantic illusion and in despair over their uncertain future, they sink into depression and may end up committing suicide. Since it is a case of emotional needs, logic or reason has no place in the search for a favorable alternative. For parents, the most appropriate behavior to solve this type of emotional conflict is to act with equanimity, without opposing the relationship, and giving the couple time to mature emotionally. Any kind of open opposition is counterproductive. As time goes by, emotions will lose some intensity and allow people to change gradually as they learn to see beyond the boundaries of their immediate environment.

The loving experience is a learning experience that develops in a progressive manner and gives us time to withdraw or change the rules of the game in case we realize that what we are involved in is in fact a false love.

LOVE AND SEX

The confusion that arises with respect to the interaction between love and sex is due mainly to our misuse of the terms and meanings relating to sex. According to the anthropological view of love, this is a biological need encoded in our genes and internal chemistry, with the brain as the anatomical substratum of its physiology and expression. True love involves sexual intimacy. For this reason it is part of the human instinct for reproduction and conservation. But no matter how strong the sexual impulse, it is not the same as love. It is part of love. "To make love" and "to have sex" are different in meaning, even though both involve intercourse. We must bear in mind that humans are the only species that engages in sexual intercourse as a source of pleasure. What "making love" and "having sex" have in common is the experience of physical pleasure. We have distinguished between the two when we talked about the erotic experience. Making love is a deeper experience in which the sexual act entails an intense and reciprocal emotional relation between a man and a woman involving not only the physical aspect but also the psychological component expressed by feelings, desires, sensations, and fantasies. Making love may or may not include the purpose of conception. It is essentially a relationship in which the man and the woman participate by mutual consent under the attraction of a shared emotional drive to achieve physical and emotional fulfillment. Having sex lacks these properties. It may be based on violence and submission of one of the parties, normally the woman. In married life, having sexual intercourse is not always equivalent to "making love." It is common for the wife to participate in the sexual act just to satisfy the husband. She may pretend to participate and even simulate an orgasm so as not to disappoint her husband.

If a woman has never had an orgasm, she cannot simulate it, since the muscle contractions are involuntary and they involve the simultaneous operation of several muscles. If the man knows something about the physiology of female orgasm and has experienced it before, he will notice when it does not happen.

If this occurs frequently, it leads to a difficult situation when the woman later decides to seek professional help as to how to achieve orgasm. It is a negative and destructive experience. It is also inappropriate to call "lover" the person with whom one has sexual relations. To characterize that person as "a great lover" can only mean that he or she is a sex machine, and acrobat, an athlete in physical terms, not somebody that really knows how to love better than others. The expression "consummating the sexual act" is also misleading since it implies that the first sexual encounter makes the interpersonal relationship somehow complete. In fact many of the relationships based on false love end soon after "consummation." The course of true love has nothing to do with whether one has had sex or not. Yet many naïve people think that "having sex" and "making love" are similar, and that a well executed sexual act reflects the quality and degree of love, and that sex is the primary component of a loving relationship. This confusion between sex and love is most common among women, who conclude that "we sleep together, so we must be in love." When sex is exciting in a relationship, both men and women may fall into the false perception that excellent sex is equivalent to true love. Sex is a basic human instinct, and lust and pleasure are the tools for its satisfaction. For many reasons, including basic physiology, conditioning, and hormones, men are in general more driven by pleasure and lust than women.

Hormones play an important role in sexual behavior. The hormonal disparity between men and women is most noticeable in young people. Male hormones at this age are very potent, and young men tend to be driven more by lust than by love. They are susceptible not only to peer pressure but also pressure from their fathers, who want them to prove their masculinity, so they are encouraged to engage in sex at an early age. For many adult males who are insecure in other areas, sexual activity is a means of building up their ego. In these cases, sex has more to do with self-love than with love for others. It provides a means of validating that partially compensates for frustrations and failures in other areas.

For men, the likelihood of confusion between love and sex is not as great as for women. However, men are more likely to fall in love under the spell of an exciting sexual experience. Women are less susceptible to use sex for self-gratification, but they are not immune to it. They may have trouble accepting that their passion is based on pleasure or lust, but they take particular pride in seducing men and making them fall in love with them. Women who have been taught that it is shameful to feel pleasure tend to emphasize the dignity of love. Men keep track of how many women they have slept with, while women are concerned with how many men have fallen in love with them.

Sexual activity is just one of the many aspects of true love, and it is possible to love someone without there being a sexual component. Sexual intimacy is as powerful as it is emotional and physically beneficial. It is a necessity for most couples that love each other. In true love, a satisfactory sexual relationship is the gradual result of the harmonious evolution of the interpersonal relationship. The deeper and more complex the couple's interaction becomes, the better their sexual relationship.

Even though sexually activity is very important, it cannot be the only basis for interpersonal relationships. Sexual activity is not a barometer of love, but only of the moment. The quality of sexual interaction changes drastically with each individual's level of desire, as well as with worries, anxiety, health, drugs, and alcohol. What matters is to enjoy sex when it is satisfying and to accept honestly that there will be times when it will not be optimally so.

In the course of an interpersonal relationship, it is not always easy to decide when to initiate sexual activity. If the only goal of the relationship is to have sex, there is no need to wait very long, but if the purpose is to develop a loving relationship, it may be a mistake to have sex on the first or second date. In any case, it may be dangerous, due to the high risk of catching a sexually transmitted disease unless one adopts the necessary precautions. Whether to wait for a week or a year will depend on common sense, mutual trust and the wishes of the interested parties. Common sense suggests that one should achieve a certain degree of emotional and mental intimacy with one's partner before trying to establish sexual intimacy. Consequently it is important to get to know each other and take time to build mutual trust, to develop closeness as a person before trying to establish physical closeness. It may be hard to remember this under the influence of a strong attraction, but trust takes time to build in any relationship. One learns to trust and have faith in another person by observing how he or she treats us or others in different levels of intimacy and how he or she operates emotionally and intellectually. This requires extensive discussion, sharing of experiences and attitudes toward sexuality and love, and making sure that there is mutual acceptance of each other's priorities.

Teenagers tend to misinterpret what love and sex really mean, whether intentionally or not. It is usually the young man who, partly because of hormones, partly because of peer pressure, initiates a behavioral pattern aimed at obtaining erotic satisfaction. He puts pressure on his partner to go along with the idea that consummating the sexual act is a demonstration of how much she loves him. The rejection of this pressure may lead to the end of the relationship.

On the other hand, we must keep in mind that teenage girls will act and dress provocatively in order to attract the attention of the most popular young man, thus satisfying their ego and earning the admiration of their rivals. It is crucial that both the young man and the young woman be aware of the potential dangers they expose themselves to. They must consider whether or not they have enough biological and emotional maturity to consummate the sexual act. This seems like a reasonable and practical consideration, but it is difficult because emotions interfere with our capacity to analyze our behavior logically. Communication and advice from the parents are very important for preventing grave consequences. Teenagers should have at least some basic information to prevent unwanted pregnancies or the transmission of a sexual disease.

What is the young person's responsibility with respect to these consequences? What will be the effect on the young woman's dignity once the momentary passion is over? If the couple is unable to prevent the consummation of the sexual act, did he use any protection or did she use any contraceptives? Are they capable of considering future consequences and responsibilities? What will be the repercussions on their ability to complete their education and professional training? What will be the emotional impact on their parents? These questions must be considered. The most serious damage will no doubt be for the young woman.

She will suffer the negative effects of a sense of guilt and depression, after the sexual act has been consummated, whether she engaged in it voluntarily or under pressure. It is possible that, even though all precautions are taken, the change will not be significant in the short term, because human nature is such that changing one's sexual behavior takes time. During the last 40 or 50 years, there have been over a million teenage pregnancies per year.

It is not surprising then that abandoned babies are found every day in diverse and unimaginable places. There has also been an increase in venereal diseases among teenagers.

There are laws, at least in Texas, that prevent the prosecution of mothers who, instead of abandoning their babies, leave them in charge of hospitals, nurses or doctors.

Love

DEFINITION

Love must be defined with respect to the specific person or being who is the object of our affection. Different manifestations of this affective state are love of God, love of nature, of life, of family, of art, self love, Platonic love, etc. As can be seen from these examples, the term "love" is used in a very general and flexible manner. It is harder to define it in a more restricted and specific fashion. By love of God we designate a religious sentiment. Love of nature, life, family, country, or art is a special feeling that involves affection, loyalty, or a deep interest. Its definition is captured by what people generally understand it to mean: a special affection or feeling.

The existence of love is universally accepted. What we are interested in here is the definition of love in an interpersonal relationship. Its origin, evolution, and the way it has been encoded in our brains are matters of keen interest that deserve special attention, since love is what attracts, selects, and unites the partners in a couple. Some of the questions that need an answer are: How does love arise or establish itself?; What is its biological foundation?; What is its anatomical and physiological substratum?; What are the factors that trigger it?

SCIENTIFIC RESEARCH

Despite the fact that love is the most intense emotion in a couple's relationship, it has not been the object of intense scientific study. A lot more attention has been paid to emotions like fear and rage, because their physical manifestations, such as pulse rate, breathing, and muscular contractions are easily measured in the laboratory. This cannot be done with love. Fear and rage bear directly on the survival of the species: the fight-and-flee reaction. It is incorrect to confuse love with the sexual instinct, since the goal of the latter, namely reproduction, can be met without any love at all.

As a result of the spread of AIDS caused by casual sexual encounters, there has been a new interest in the scientific study of love. The importance of knowing more about this force that keeps couples together has been acknowledged. Another factor is the increasing number of female scientists who have shown more interest than their male counterparts in the serious study of love. Whatever the reason, the fact is that science has come to acknowledge something that is universally accepted: love is real, not just a fantasy, and is part of our biology.

SOCIO-CULTURAL EVOLUTION

It is important to know the socio-cultural influence of love. It has been said that if love did not exist there would not be any poets or novelists. For them love is ecstasy and torture, freedom and slavery, and it keeps the world turning. Around the 12th century the troubadours from Provence invented the Art of Courtly Love, a very elaborate ritual for noble ladies of leisure wanting to experience love who would have been scandalized by any insinuation of sexual consummation. Ever since, the ideas of love and being loved have been a dominant theme of popular culture as expressed in music, films, novels, magazines and a great part of what is seen on television. Love is powerful and it has proved to be a commercial commodity: people buy whatever promises them the happiness of romance. The psychologist Lawrence Casher, author of Is Matrimony Necessary?, has said that love is a fake emotion that we accept because our culture celebrates it. He furthermore does not believe that love is part of human nature but a consequence of social pressure, and concludes by stating that even if it were part of human nature, like crime or violence, it is not necessarily desirable.

The prevailing idea, according to Darwin's theory, is that reproduction is the main motivation for sex. Why is it then that love is part of the process, since it was presumably not necessary for sex? Furthermore, what accounts for love's persistence through centuries? What is its motivating impulse?

When we analyze love rationally, we see that people in love state that love gives them energy and makes them feel attracted and spellbound. If love were pure fiction with no perceptible and rational evidence, most people would surely be immune to it. But this is not what has happened. Love is still in the air and has probably spread more than even romantics would have imagined. Those who think love is a cultural fantasy have been influenced by the viewpoint of certain social classes in 12th century central Europe. According to them love arises thanks to the refinements peculiar to Western culture. The availability of free time, leisure, a comfortable life, a certain refinement in the arts and literature favor the development of love among members of the aristocracy. Hence the saying that aristocrats fall in love and peasants just mate.

The anthropologists William Jankowick and Edward Fischer have found evidence of romantic love in 147 out of 166 primitive cultures they studied. These findings make it clear that love is not an invention of Western culture but a biological fact. Love, which can be found in many cultures, is a universal phenomenon common to all humanity, although not everybody expresses it the same way. The fact that in a particular culture love is not expressed by dimmed lights, background music, and pretty bouquets of flowers does not mean that it does not exist. The anthropologist Helen Fischer says she never imagined that love was such a primitive human emotion, like fear, rage or pleasure. The problem is that anthropologists have looked for love in the wrong social contexts, mainly courting and wedding rituals. In many cultures matrimony and love do not go together; matrimony is more like the merger of two corporations signed and approved by the couple's families to protect their territorial interests.

BIOLOGICAL CONSIDERATIONS

Many scientists believe that the biological predisposition to love is encoded in our genes and internal chemistry. What remains to be explored is the ways that humans have chosen to express this emotional aspect of their lives. According to these considerations there is evidence that love is solidly based on the biological and chemical evolution of neurotransmitters. What appears irrational in the surface observation of lovers' behavior is part of the master strategy of nature, a vital force that has allowed humans to survive, prosper and multiply through millennia.

It is believed that love started to flourish in Africa about four million years ago with the beginning of the human species, as neurotransmitters began to flow in blood vessels producing the awkward facial expressions and sweaty palms that men and women experience as they make eye contact. As humanity evolved and man stopped walking an all fours and adopted an erect position, the whole body became more visible for his peers. His genitalia, the color of his eyes, the breadth of his shoulders, were thus fully exhibited for the first time. As never before, each individual had unique attractive characteristics. This provides new avenues that allow the sexual instinct to attain a romantic encounter and not just be a reproductive act. Human beings, unlike animals, began to enjoy face-to-face copulation, and attraction became an important factor for couples. This way love has served the evolutionary purpose of keeping man and woman together for a long period of time, which is essential for raising children. Primitive couples stayed together for just enough time to allow the development of their child until his or her early teens. Then, each member looked for a new partner to start the process all over again. This cycle was repeated at least every four years, a phenomenon that Helen Fisher refers to as "the four-year itch." According to her studies, statistics reveal a high incidence of divorce precisely according to this pattern. In most of the 62 cultures studied by this anthropologist, divorce is very high around the fourth year of matrimony. Young couples may stay together longer, and the birth of a second child may prolong the union for another four years.

If love is a natural disposition, it is neither eternal nor exclusive. Less than 5% of mammals form strictly faithful couples. The human model has been monogamy with clandestine adultery. Men looked for new partners to have more children. Contrary to common belief, women also showed this tendency but kept their extramarital relations secret. They would go behind the bushes with their secret lovers, and this way they unknowingly transmitted through the centuries the characteristics of the female soul that make modern women adept at flirting. Infidelity has always existed; it is not an exclusive behavior of modern times.

Lovers often claim that there is a strong power that produces mutual attraction. According to researchers, what happens is a complex neurochemical cascade. Looking into each other's eyes, touching hands, the perception of a perfume, the very presence of the other person, all this can trigger stimuli that starts in the brain and is transmitted through the blood stream to the different nerve terminals.

The results of this stimulation are well known: blushing, sweating, and accelerated breathing. In this sense, love is very much like stress, since the neurochemical mechanisms are the same. We should not be surprised either by the lovers' expression of happiness and euphoria, given the number of neurotransmitting substances at play, mainly dopamine and norepinephrine, derived from phenylalanine. In this respect love is a natural euphoria. This state, triggered by dopamine and phenylalanine, is not permanent, and that is why passionate love does not last very long. It is believed that the human organism develops immunity to phenylalanine and that its levels may vary. After two or three years, the amount of phenylalanine produced by the organism decreases and this marks the end of the relationship. It may be that factors other than neurotransmitters may intervene and extend the duration of love. It is also believed that other neurotransmitters associated with endorphins may play a role. These are substances produced in specific areas of the brain that control our perception of pain. Their effect is very similar to that of morphine, which produces a sense of wellbeing, calm, and security. This may account in part for our sense of despair when we are abandoned or our loved one dies. According to researchers, there is a clear contrast between the passion induced by the phenylalanine derivatives and the more intimate and lasting affective relationship triggered by endorphins.

There is another chemical substance produced by the brain and recently associated with love, oxytocin, which sensitizes nerve terminals and stimulates muscle contractions. In women, this substance plays a role in the contraction of the uterus during childbirth, it stimulates milk production, and it seems to inspire mothers to coddle their babies. Some scientists believe that oxytocin might strengthen petting among adult lovers, facilitate erection, and intensify orgasm.

ANATOMICAL BASIS OF LOVE

We have so far discussed the neurochemical foundation of love. These considerations lead us to the anatomical substratum that underlies them. The different neurochemical substances produced by the brain are mediated by the central nervous system.

Love is an emotion that, like fear or anger, has an organic foundation. An emotion is a condition of the organism that reveals itself in bodily changes, mainly visceral, under the control of the autonomous nervous system, and in association with a mental state of excitement or disturbance leading to a specific type of behavior. Happiness, love, hate, and fear are examples of primary emotions. Anxiety and sadness are secondary emotions with a lower degree of visceral reaction.

The cerebral mechanisms that control emotions are located in the limbic system, which includes the middle sections of the temporal, frontal and parietal lobes with their central connections to the cerebral tonsil, the septal region, the pre-optical area, the hypothalamus, the anterior thalamus, the habenula, and the central tegument of the middle brain. The peripheral nervous system consists of the autonomous nervous system and the visceral structures under its control. For a better understanding of the importance of the normal function of the center of emotions we will describe in general the studies and disorders of the better-known emotions, some of which are to some extent related to the process of love.

EMOTIONAL INSTABILITY

Emotional reactions of babies and children are easily triggered because of their inability to inhibit them. Control of one's emotions is gradually acquired through maturation of the brain, learning, satisfaction of one's needs, and social conditioning. The process of growing up includes the acquisition of the ability to inhibit our emotions, which does not mean that their intensity decreases but rather that we gain control over them to the point of being able to suppress their manifestation.

The expression of emotions among adults varies not only between men and women but also between different cultures. Emotional reactions that are permissible in one culture may not be in a different one.

Individuals who have suffered severe brain damage may lose the ability to control their emotions. In these cases a small stimulus may provoke an emotional reaction. The emotional reaction expressed primarily by tears and loud and prolonged laughter may be triggered by a mildly comical situation, the re encounter with an old acquaintance, or even just somebody singing the national anthem. What these cases have in common is the lack of proportion between the stimulus and the reaction, although the expression may be proportionate to the visceral and motor components of the emotional state.

This condition may also be observed in a milder way among older individuals, probably due to vascular insufficiency in the brain. Needless to say, this can be embarrassing for the person in question.

EXPLOSIVE LAUGHTER AND CRYING

These individuals, due to a brain disorder, undergo episodes or crises of incontrollable explosive laughter and crying that are easily triggered and can last several minutes. This can lead to exhaustion if the crisis is prolonged. Normally emotional reaction and affection are consistent with the situation that provokes them. Explosive laughter and crying are pathological because the reaction is always incommensurate with the stimulus and there is no possibility of moderation, whether the expression is of pleasure or sadness. The mechanism of emotional inhibition simply does not exist. This condition is often the result of pseudo-bulbar paralysis, a lesion of the cerebral stem distal segment, whose function it is to control the components of facial muscles, respiratory functions, and visceral muscles.

AGGRESSIVENESS, VIOLENCE, ANGER, RAGE, AND FURY

This set of emotional reactions is particularly important not only in interpersonal relations but also in romantic relations. Primary emotions in a sublimated form may be acceptable as patterns of social behavior. Tantrums, reactions of incontrollable anger or rage in a less sublimated fashion are accepted in sporting competitions (boxing, American football, basketball, hockey, etc.). In a modified form we see them in scholastic competitions and in daring and audacious business transactions. The degree of evolution that must be achieved in order for these primary reactions of violence and aggressiveness to be more subtle varies from one individual to another. There are significant differences between men and women. Hormones and physical characteristics make men much more aggressive than women. This process, particularly in men, is not completed until age 25 or 30, sometimes even later. The persistence of this type of emotional reaction constitutes an abnormal sociopathic behavior. Individuals in this condition may at the slightest provocation change from a calm state to one of wild rage and blind impulses towards violence and destruction. They completely lose touch with reality and are totally impermeable to any reasoning or pleading. Once the crisis is over, some will show remorse over what they have done. What is obviously abnormal is the strength or degree of the aggressive reaction, totally out of proportion to the insignificance of the stimulus that provoked it. The study of this type of individuals highlights the importance of developing a normal emotional behavior.

This type of emotional reaction must be modified through the individual's development so as transform it and channel it into feelings of tolerance and respect. The natural place for this transformation to occur is home. The most influential role models for the child have always been and continue to be the child's parents. The plasticity of a child's brain makes it possible to learn the appropriate social attitudes and behaviors that will enable the child in the future to establish stable and lasting interpersonal relationships. We must live our lives according to the highest standards of ethical behavior, since this is what out children and our community expect of us. The harmony, tolerance, respect, consideration, appreciation and affection exhibited by the parents will affect the normal development of an adult personality. Studies on domestic violence show that people with an aggressive personality have been raised in a broken family environment and have been deprived of the most basic affection required by a mind in the process of maturation and development.

INDIFFERENCE AND APATHY

Most patients with brain damage experience a quantitative reduction in all psychomotor activities. Both their thoughts and their words and movements are impaired. This motor deficiency is also manifested in conversation, which reveals a lack of continuous psychic activity, slowness of thought, and a diminished perception, curiosity, and interest in the patient's surroundings. There is also a deficient threshold of stimulation; attention is inconsistent and incapable of focusing and maintaining alertness, and there is apathy and lack of initiative (abulia).

ALTERATIONS OF SEXUALITY

The normal patterns of sexual behavior may be altered as a result of lesions in the limbic system. Lesions in the orbital sections of the frontal lobes may cause the elimination of ethical and moral restrictions and are associated with indiscriminate hypersexuality. Injury to the superior pre-frontal areas of the brain may produce abulia, lack of initiative and sexual drive, and it may also affect other functions. Sexual hyperactivity has been observed in men and women with encephalitis and tumors in the temporal lobe. Stimulation of the septal ventral area causes sensations of pleasure and lust. There has also been observed an awakening of sexual drive in epileptic patients exhibiting psychomotor attacks affecting the middle face of the temporal lobe. A diminished libido and sexuality are common manifestations of depression. On the other hand, most epileptics with lesions in other areas of the temporal lobe exhibit a greatly reduced sexual activity.

The importance of knowing about alterations of sexuality related to certain brain injuries lies in their participation in the emotions that accompany these alterations. Anxiety, fear, and depression are affective manifestations that interfere with the stability of interpersonal and romantic relationships.

SOCIO-CULTURAL ASPECTS

The influence of socio-cultural factors during the growing years, coupled with the maturation of the nervous system, is important for the modulation and expression of emotions. As a consequence, love cannot but be conditioned somehow by the individual's parents and socio-cultural environment.

Even though we do not fully understand its intrinsic mechanisms, it is a fact that love is an emotion that has a biological basis. Its expression throughout the centuries adopts different forms, according to the cultural characteristics of each society.

Love plays a crucial role in the selection of partners. Men look for fertility, so women between the ages of 17 and 28 are the most desirable. Men have the ability to evaluate youth and vitality with just one look. They fall in love easily. Women, on the other hand, do it more slowly because their requirements are more complex. They need more time to study a man. Age may not be a crucial factor, but women look for a man who can provide security, be the father of their children, have a certain social status and sufficient economic resources.

The selection of a particular person, according to the sexologist John Money, is determined by each individual's characteristics, a set of features that he refers to as a "love map". This map is the result personal characteristics and childhood experiences. It constitutes a register of what we find exciting and seductive, what does not bother or irritate us. All the information acquired during our growing years is imprinted in our brain circuitry. When a sufficient number of these characteristics match those of another person, a connection is established that may facilitate a reaction of love.

All human beings have the potential to love. As children we learn to feel loved by our parents and from them we learn to love others. If we do not experience love as children it becomes harder to love in the future. That is why there are people who spend their whole lives searching for love without finding it. Family is our first social world. If the family functions harmoniously and we feel our parents' love and affection, we will learn what love is without explicit instruction. Later, when we start school, we enter a new social and cultural environment whose influence we cannot escape, although the strongest influence will no doubt be that of our family. At school it will be up to our teachers to teach us how to love, and we will only learn the type of love that they themselves have internalized. If the type of love they learned is immature and exclusive, that is what they teach their students. If, on the other hand, they have learned that love is free, mature and that it evolves, that is what they will teach. Language is the main way of transmitting knowledge, attitudes, prejudices, feelings, and whatever makes personalities and cultures unique. Language is very important for the establishment of behavior, relationships, attitudes, empathy, responsibility, attention, happiness, and the capacity to react; in other words, to establish what we might call the language of love.

Through education young people get their first exposure to a new and wide world full of different, exceptional, and exciting attitudes towards life and love. Unfortunately they are disillusioned very shortly. Rather than feeling free to make their own way, they find that the new environment is even less flexible than home. The school experience follows a rigid obligatory path dictated by law. Formal education takes its main function to be the continuation of the knowledge accumulated in the past, often at the expense of the present and future. Young people are taught everything except what they need for their development as individuals and in relation to others. The current educational system teaches neither love of self nor love of others. As a result the individual, now fully developed, leaves school in a state of confusion, loneliness, alienation, and irritation, but with the mind full of meaningless isolated facts, what we laughably call an education.

We can conclude that formal education does not teach us to love. At no point during the educational process are young people exposed to love as a subject of study. Whatever they have learned about love they have acquired indirectly and haphazardly. Their main source of information has been the commercial media, which have always exploited love for their own purposes. So the home environment is the only place that can offer young people an example of true love as long as the interpersonal relations between parents and children are favorable and operate within a sincere, spontaneous, and objective framework.

What we learn in school is friendship and camaraderie, not because of formal instruction but by osmosis through group activities such as sports, the boy scouts, or social events like music, dancing, and the theatre, plus religious or other family functions. Love is a vital human necessity from childhood through all the different stages of development. It is a biological imperative without which humans cannot survive. During their first years, children are totally defenseless and need the attention and care of their elders, particularly their parents. Without close links of human interaction the newly born may in fact retrogress in its development. Research has shown that children are more adversely affected by their parents' divorce, separation or death than by illness or any combination of other factors. There are several studies that point to a positive correlation between affection and togetherness on the one hand and growth and development on the other. Children may seem not to understand the subtle dynamics of love, yet they have a strong need for it that can affect their future development. This need does not change as the child becomes a teenager and an adult. In many cases the need for love and togetherness is the main force in young people's or adult's loving relationships. During puberty, when young people start relating to each other, parents often make mistakes, especially when dates are frequent or prolonged. Since such dates may involve problems, parents must communicate wit their children directly, not through coercive measures. During puberty young people are undergoing specific hormonal changes. The initial caresses and kisses, which may be innocent, start intensifying and may awaken sensations and emotions that may culminate in the consummation of the sexual act.

It is at this stage and circumstances that parents' intervention must be made with clarity and understanding. First, parents must respect the existence of their children's relations, whether they like them or not. Second, they must explain to their children that their behavior may lead to consequences that should be avoided. The consummation of the sexual act may, on the one hand, lead to an unexpected and undesired pregnancy, and on the other, to the possibility of contracting a sexually transmitted disease. Young people undergoing puberty are not in a position to assume the responsibility of a casual sexual encounter. Consciously or not, the young man, driven by instinct, wants his partner to acknowledge this drive as a sign of love. The young woman who gives in spite of her parents' advice is acting not only incorrectly but also immorally. Knowing that her resistance may lead to the termination of the relationship, she may give in and then be faced with strong emotional reactions, such as a sense of guilt and shame. This reaction becomes more dramatic if she gets pregnant. The young man has two options: accept responsibility or break the relationship. The latter is the most likely outcome. If the young man accepts his responsibility, the problems and requirements of this new facet of the relationship may be emotionally and financially devastating. This might be averted through understanding and help from the parents. Whatever the case, the ensuing coexistence will not have the romance that they could have experienced if they had the strength to wait until they matured psychologically and biologically.

If, on the other hand, the young woman does not go along with her partner's urging, the relationship may come to an end. This outcome will cause pain when she realizes that her true love and honorable behavior were not appreciated. This might lead to disappointment and depression and to future rejections or sexual lack of satisfaction.

In the first case, when the young woman yields to avoid rejection, she will eventually be abandoned anyway. I have observed this repeatedly among fourteen or fifteen year old girls who got pregnant under pressure by their partners on the erroneous belief that they were demonstrating their true love or for fear of being abandoned.

As we said before, sex is not love; it is part of love when the latter exists between emotionally and biologically mature people who are aware of the consequences of sex and of the responsibility they assume when they practice it. But mature couples are not immune to the problems that affect younger people. In some cases a single woman leaves home because the situation is unbearable due to affective and/or economic reasons. Lack of parental affection or conflict between mother and father force women, more often than men, to seek independence. This separation may be beneficial, but in some cases it may be disastrous. The woman may take the first opportunity to enter into a relationship. Quite often, she will look for someone resembling her father both in positive and in negative qualities. This is most likely when the young woman has received more affection from her father than from her mother. The reverse is the case for young men. If a young man is emotionally closer to his mother than to his father, he will chose a partner that resembles his mother and that will often be older than him.

Love is not eternal, in spite of what we promise each other at the start of a loving relationship. Love is an emotional state with high and low points and varying duration. The flame that feeds passion at the beginning gradually fades and eventually dies. Caresses and dedication to each other are not what they used to be. We forget important dates, our wedding anniversary, our partner's birthday, that special romantic dinner by candlelight, the birth of our first child, etc.

True love eventually becomes friendship, camaraderie, mutual support, participation in mutually pleasing activities, harmonious coexistence, sharing rough hours or days, solving the problems inherent to human existence with honest and spontaneous communication.

Love and a satisfying erotic relation is no guarantee either that the couple will stay together for a long time. A satisfying sexual relation is not necessarily permanent, just like love. There are biological and hormonal factors that can have a negative impact on both men and women, not to mention illness and medicine used for medical treatment. Since man has the more active role in sex, these factors are noticed first in him, and the woman may interpret the change as lack of love, infidelity, or absence of physical attraction.

If the couple is not aware of the factors that affect the development and evolution of human sexuality, the consequences are generally detrimental for a sustained coexistence. Under these conditions, erotic play may be just as satisfying as the sexual act. Love is not unique. Both men and women may fall in love with more than one person. It all depends of the circumstances and the opportunities available. Love may come to an end after either a short or a long period of coexistence if it is not complemented with the factors responsible for the stability of interpersonal relationships described in the relevant preceding chapters.

The Erotic Experience

When we talk about the sexual experience we normally associate it with the physical aspect of intercourse. Strictly speaking, only vaginal penetration by the penis qualifies as "sexual relation". Any other modality of erotic stimulation is just another expression of human sexuality. The erotic experience includes both a physical and a psychological component. The expressions "to have sex" or "to make love" point quite clearly to the difference we want to establish between sexual relation and erotic experience.

Biologically, the aim of sexual relations is procreation, reproduction and preservation of the human species. Both for humans and other animals, sexual relation is part of their conservation instinct. On the other hand, when we talk about "erotic experience" we are dealing with something broader between a man and a woman that includes feelings, desires, sensations and fantasies. Participation in the erotic experience is not limited to physical pleasure; it also encompasses the emotional satisfaction that comes from communicating one's feelings, from mutual possession, from love and tenderness. When the interpersonal relation is positive there is an intense and mutual emotional exchange. Unfortunately, if the interpersonal relation is negative there cannot be an erotic experience. The couple may "have sex" under these circumstances, but without any mutual emotional involvement. When the interpersonal relation is negative, one of the parties engages in sex solely so that his or her partner can get sexual satisfaction. Normally it is the woman who surrenders physically so that the man can be satisfied. She may fake an orgasm to give the impression that she is also being satisfied. It is less common that the man would go through the motions to satisfy his partner because if he is not aroused he is likely not to get an adequate erection or to have a premature ejaculation. If a man is not acquainted with the physical manifestation of female orgasm, he may be fooled into thinking that he has satisfied his partner. This cycle may be repeated frequently, leaving him with the impression that he has "made love" when all he has done is to "have sex". This has serious implications when the woman seeks a solution to the problem and is reluctant to undergo therapy because she knows she has been lying and faking orgasm. Another aspect of this problem comes from participation in the sexual act under threat, that is, sexual abuse. This kind of experience is psychologically devastating for the woman that has been subjected to it. For the man, it is an expression of hostility, anger, aggressiveness, and feelings of dominance and revenge. He is more likely to engage in this behavior because of his active physical participation. But the same psychological factors may cause the woman to be passive-aggressive by showing indifference, frigidity, or offensive language, so as to demean the man's self image.

A positive erotic experience is the only way a couple can express their emotions and share the sense of pleasure associated with it. The emotional, romantic, sentimental component (or however you want to call it) is best expressed through love play prior to intercourse. Caresses, tactile or oral stimulation of different parts of the body, including sexual organs, are the physical expression of the spiritual motivation that leads both parties to an erotic union. We must keep in mind that tactile stimulation is one on the most effective means of expressing affection. The skin is used to being the receptor of caresses and affection since the moment we are born. A handshake, a pat in the back, a hug are the most common expressions of our affection, and we regrettably cease to use them with our partners after years of coexistence. The erotic experience requires not only the couple's mutual, open, and spontaneous participation but also some basic knowledge of the anatomy and physiology of its sexuality. Eliminating any erroneous ideas that might have been acquired while growing up will contribute to a better understanding of sexuality.

The purpose of this book is to provide the basic information that will allow couples to achieve sexual satisfaction on a regular basis. Female orgasm is a pleasant neurophysiological sensation or climax produced by contractions and spasms or certain muscles of the pelvic area related to genital structures similar to those that occur during male ejaculation. The feeling of relaxation, pleasure and physical and emotional well-being is related to the production of endorphins that most likely starts with foreplay and sexual intercourse. A similar effect results from the production of endorphins after thirty to sixty minutes of moderate physical exercise.

Knowing how to establish a satisfactory personal relation is essential in allowing a couple to achieve a positive erotic experience that will last through their time together. This is why we have emphasized the different factors that play a role in a relationship in the preceding chapters. They constitute the basic foundation for a couple's emotional satisfaction.

Foreplay

One of the most important activities prior to intercourse is foreplay, which prepares and predisposes the couple to make love. This is particularly necessary so that the woman is stimulated and achieves the required physio-psychological preparation to actively participate in sexual intercourse. Women need at least twenty to thirty minutes of foreplay to attain a positive disposition to make love.

From the physiological point of view, foreplay involves the stimulation of the central nervous system. Its effects are manifested in psychological and physical changes. Psychologically, both the man and the woman reach a favorable disposition to accept and share expressions of affection. Physically, the skin's sensibility, blood circulation, and secretion of the sexual organs are intensified. All of this contributes to a more pleasing physical contact.

The practice of foreplay is always a signal of a harmonious interpersonal relation. Without the latter, the former does not take place. It is thus important to emphasize that couples must always practice foreplay before sexual intercourse. We have already mentioned the activities and expressions that constitute foreplay, such as caressing different parts of the body, showering together, and giving each other erotic massages.

Important though it is to practice foreplay as a prelude to sexual intercourse, it should not be limited to that function. Rather, it should be practiced any time the man and the woman are together. Foreplay thus need not be necessarily erotic. Any verbal expression or caress may have special meaning as a token of appreciation or love. What matters is that these expressions be spontaneous and not forced. To sustain foreplay, as part or lovemaking or otherwise, as we have said, requires a satisfactory and harmonious interpersonal relation.

Anatomy of the Sexual Organs

It is desirable to be acquainted with some basic facts concerning the anatomy and physiology of the male and female sexual organs. I will offer here some general information supplemented by illustrations.

THE MALE GENITALIA

The male genitalia include the testicles, the ductus deferens, the seminal vesicles, the ejaculatory ducts, the penis, and two ancillary structures: the prostate, and the bulbourethral glands (Figs. 1, 2).

The testicles are two parenchymatous organs whose function is the production of spermatozoa. They have an oval shape and are covered by a fibrous membrane called tunica albuginea. After descending from the abdominal cavity, each testicle is housed in its scrotum, a kind of sac consisting of skin and the so-called dartos tunic, located under the penis. The testicles have some mobility inside the scrotum and can ascend to the groin area by contraction of the dartos tunic, which is connected to the inguinal channel.

The internal structure of the testicles is characterized by the presence of the seminiferous tubules whose delicate walls contain different kinds of epithelial cells inside which we can see the spermatozoa in different stages of development. The seminiferous tubules converge to constitute the rete testis and then the testicular plexus that gives origin to 12 to 20 efferent ducts that exit the testicle to form the head of the epididymis, whose body and tail are located on the back side of the testicle. The ductus deferens originates at the tail of the epididymis, and from there it ascends along the internal border of the epididymis on the back side of the testicle to constitute part of the spermatic cord which ascends to the groin area and the pelvic cavity. It then continues toward the ventral side of the bladder crossing the urethra between the bladder and the internal side of the seminal vesicle, where it meets the duct from the opposite side towards the base of the prostate and joins the seminal vesicle. Due to its hard consistency, the ductus deferens may be felt with one's fingers giving the sensation of a cord. Its middle section, which is the most important, consists of muscle tissue.

The seminal vesicles are two membranous and lobe-shaped cavities located between the bottom of the bladder and the rectum. Despite their name, they do not store sperm, but produce the seminal liquid that is added to the testicular secretion at the moment of ejaculation. Their lower section is the narrowest and forms a tube that joins the one from the opposite side to constitute the ejaculatory duct, about 2 centimeters long. The ejaculatory duct starts at the base of the prostate and proceeds forward between the middle lateral lobes of the prostate narrowing down until it ends in a small orifice just between the utricle and the prostatic urethra. (Figs. 3,4,5)

The penis is attached to the front and the sides of the pubic arc. In its flaccid state it has the shape of a triangular prism with rounded angles constituting the dorsal section of the prism. It consists of three cylindrical structures of cavernous tissue connected by fibrous tissue and covered by the skin. Two of these cylindrical masses located on both sides of the penis are know as the corpora cavernosa. The third structure, located in the middle and lower part of the penis, is the corpora spongiosa. It contains most of the urethra.

The flaccid state of the penis corresponds to the period prior to sexual stimulation and after ejaculation and orgasm. There is no increased blood flow, blood pressure in the corpora cavernosa being about the same as in the veins, and there is no obstacle to the return venous flow.

In the state of tumescence, blood volume and pressure in the corpora cavernosa increase, but their dilation is not enough to interfere with the return venous flux. In the state of erection, blood flow increases rapidly so that the pressure in the corpora cavernosa augments considerably and the return venous flow is limited. This causes increased rigidity of the penis that facilitates vaginal penetration. The changes of erection disappear after ejaculation and orgasm, with the penis returning to the flaccid state previously described.

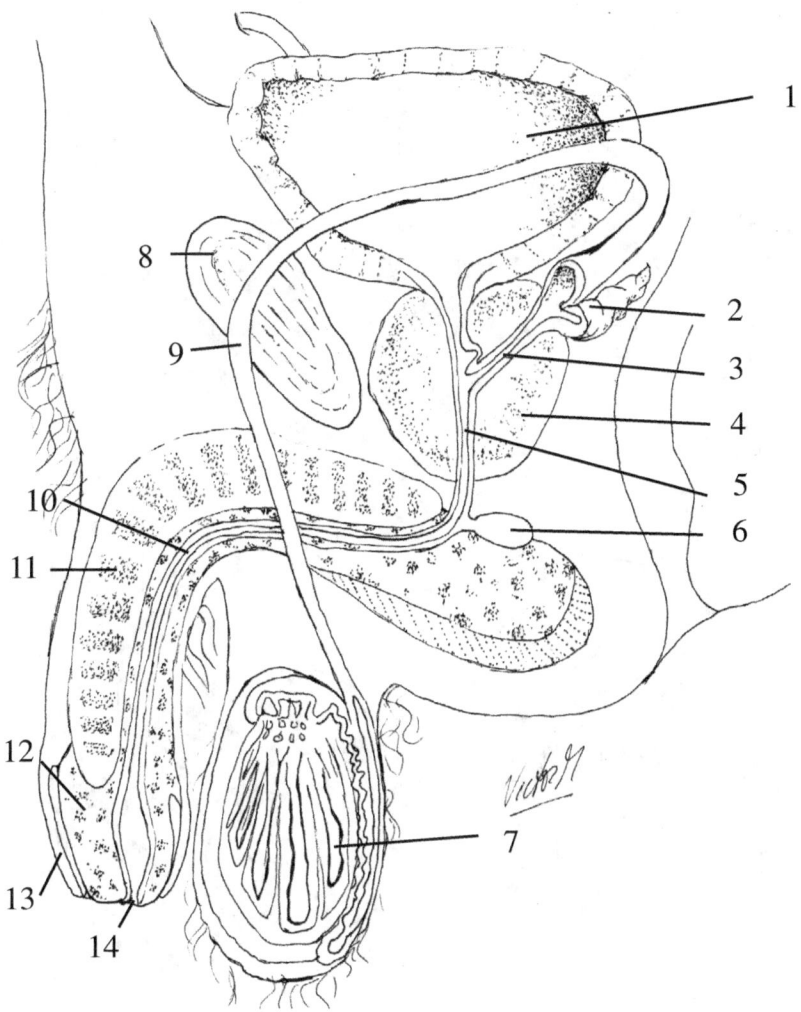

Fig. 1
Sagittal section of the male genitalia

1. Bladder, 2. Seminal vesicles, 3. Ejaculatory duct,
4. Prostate, 5. Prostatic urethra, 6. Bulbo-urethral gland,
7. Testicle, 8. Pubis, 9. Ductus deferens, 10. Urethra,
11. Corpora cavernosa, 12. Glans and corpora spongiosa,
13. Prepuce, 14. Urethral meatus.

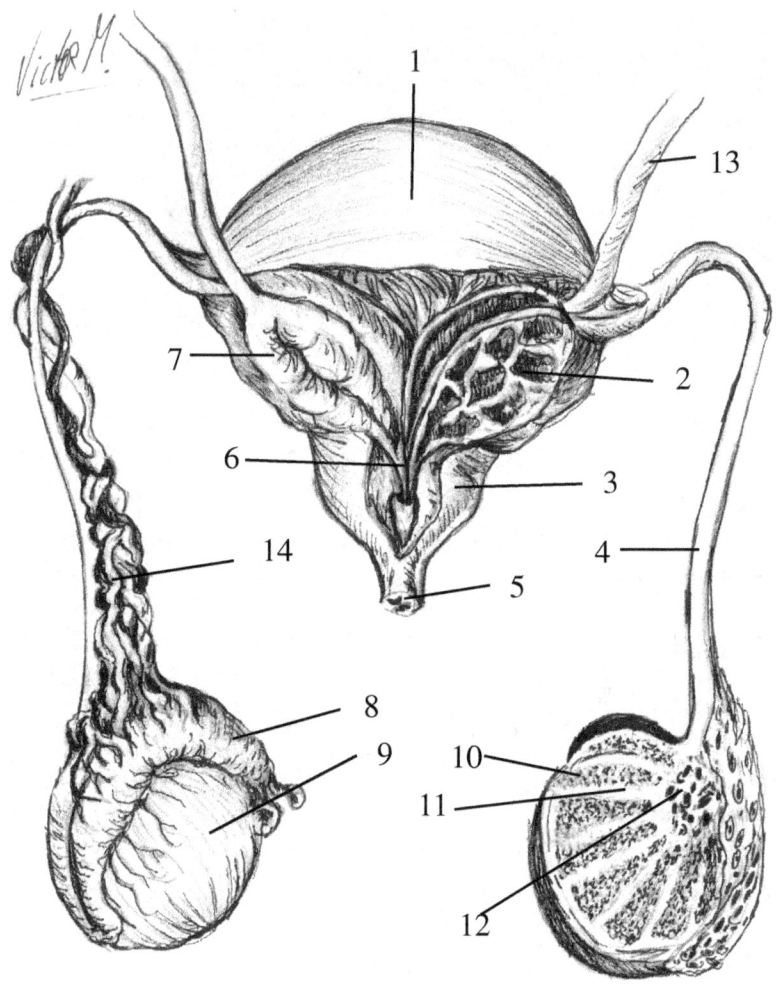

Fig. 2
Male genitalia

On right side, sagittal cut to see the internal structure
1. Bladder, 2. Seminal vesicle internal aspect, 3. Prostate,
4. Ductus deferens, 5. Urethra, 6. Ejaculatory duct, 7.Seminal
vesicle external aspect, 8. Epididymis, 9. Testicle, 10.
Testicular lobules, 11. Septum between the lobules of the
testicle, 12. Rete testis, 13. Ureter. 14. Spermatic chord.

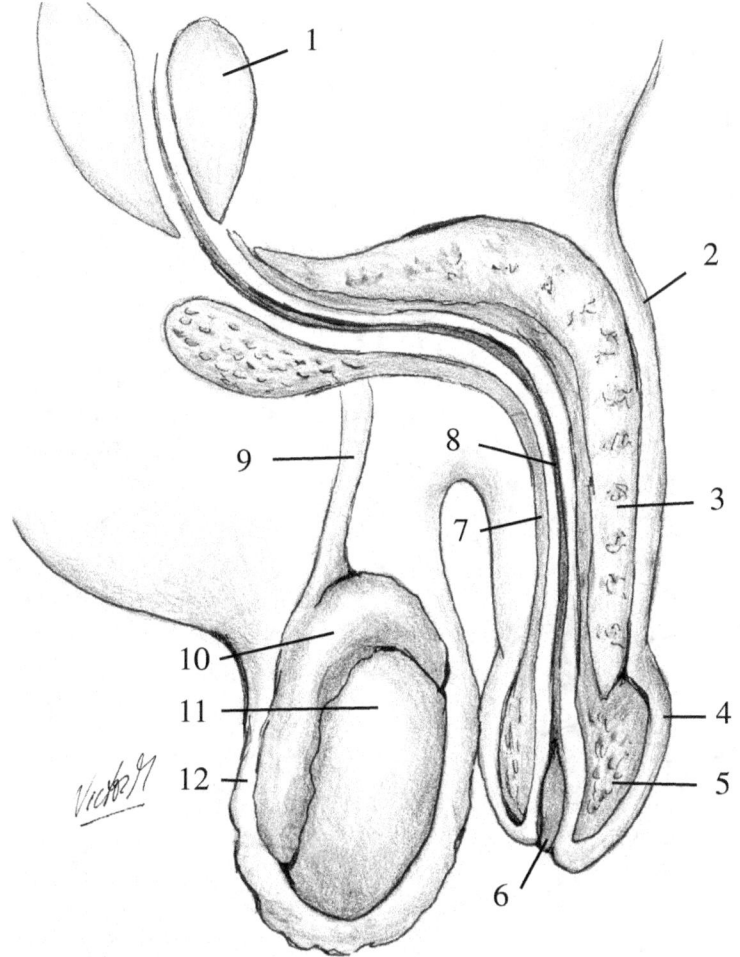

Fig. 3
Penis in flaccid state

1. Pubis, 2. Skin, 3. Corpora cavernosa with decreased intracavernosal blood pressure, 4. Prepuce, 5. Glans, 6. Urethral meatus, 7. Corpora spongiosa, 8. Urethra, 9. Spermatic chord, 10. Epididymis, 11. Testicle, 12. Scrotum.

In the resting flaccid state of the penis, the intracavernal pressure is minimal and there is no interference with venous return.

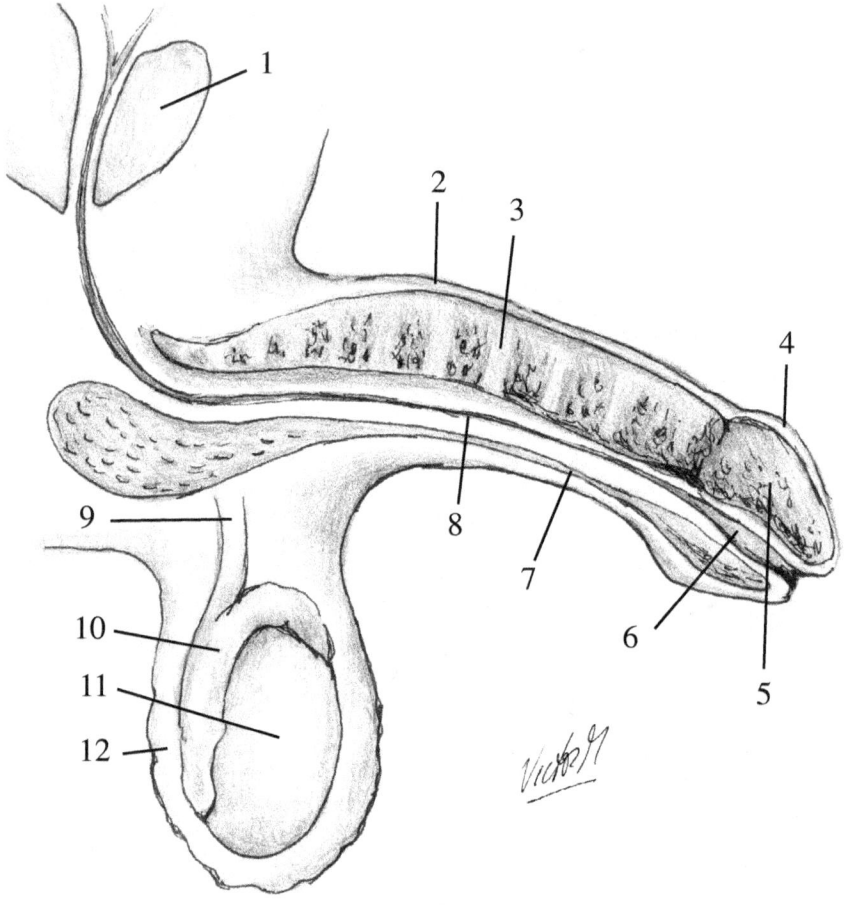

Fig. 4 Sagittal section of penis in state of tumefaction

1. Pubis, 2. Skin, 3. Corpora cavernosa of penis with slight increase of blood flow and intracavernosal pressure, 4. Prepuce, 5. Glans, 6. Urethral meatus, 7. Corpora spongiosa, 8. Urethra, 9. Spermatic chord, 10. Epididymis, 11. Testicle, 12. Scrotum.

State of penile tumefaction. There is slight increase in blood flow with partial dilatation of the corpora cavernosa and decrease of the venous blood flow.

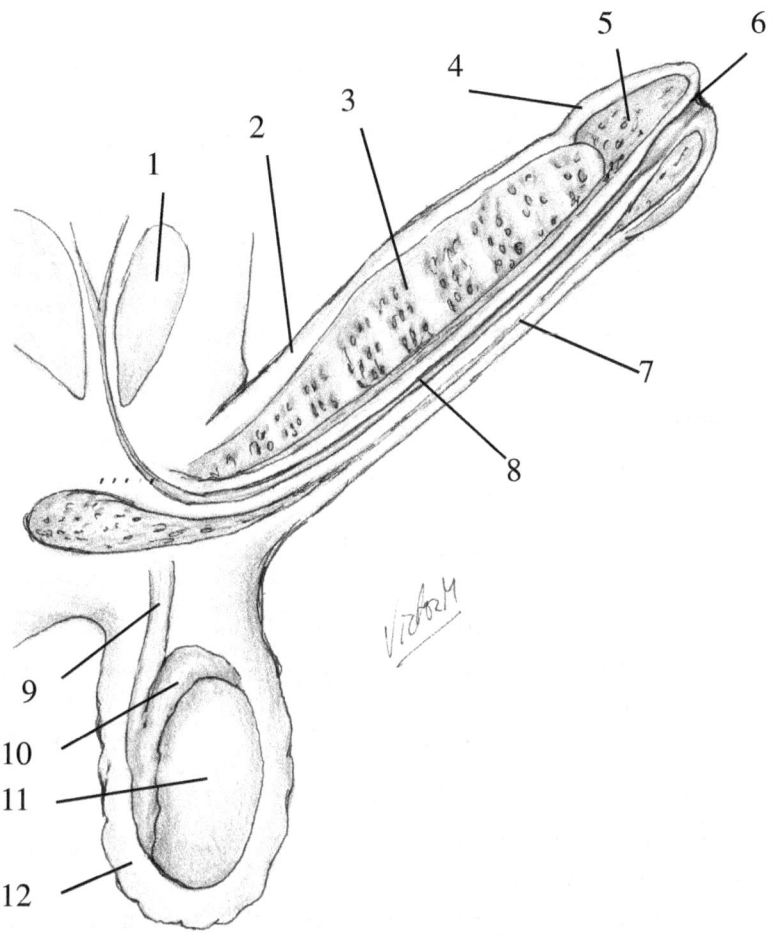

Fig.5 Sagittal section of penis in state of erection

1. Pubis, 2. Skin, 3. Corpora cavernosa with greater blood flow and increased intracavernosal pressure, 4. Prepuce, 5. Glans, 6. Urethral meatus, 7. Corpora spongiosa, 8. Urethra, 9. Spermatic chord, 10. Epididymis, 11. Testicle, 12. Scrotum.

The blood flow is increased with rapid filling and dilatation of the corpora cavernosa and marked compression of the venous system. This permits that the rigidity of the penis lasts sufficiently to allow for the execution of sex. .

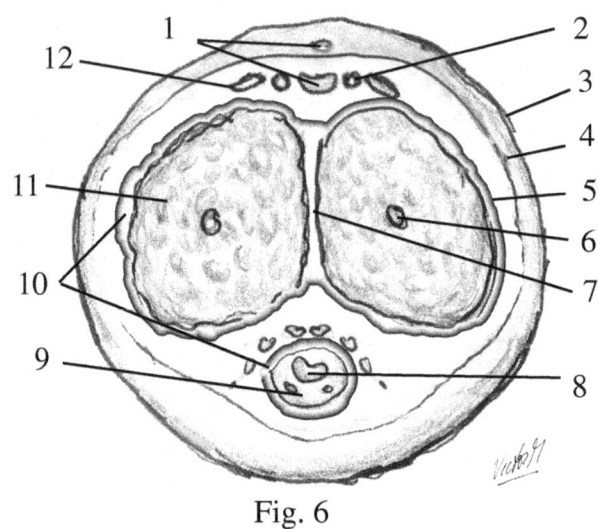

Fig. 6
Transverse section of penis

1. Superficial and deep dorsal vein, 2. Dorsal artery 3. Skin,
4. Tunica Dartos, 5. Fascia profunda of penis, 6. Central artery
of corpora cavernosa, 7. Penile septum, 8. Urethra, 9. Corpora
spongiosa, 10. Tunica Albuginea, 11. Corpora cavernosa, 12.
Dorsal nerve

With impotence of vascular origin, the flaccid state, the state of
tumescence, and the state of erection do not occur.

The skin covering the penis is very thin. It lacks adipose tissue and
it does not adhere to the structural parts of the penis. At the base of
the penis, the skin connects with the skin of the pubis, the scrotum
and the perineum. Towards the front, on the stem of the penis, the
skin separates from the surface and forms the prepuce (or foreskin).
Right after the external orifice of the urethra, the prepuce forms a
small reduplication that extends from the meatus of the urethra to
the neck of the penis forming the frenulum. On the neck of the penis
and the internal surface of the prepuce are located the preprucial
glands, which secrete a sebaceous material with a peculiar odor that
decomposes rapidly when mixed with epithelial discharges and is
called the smegma.

The internal surface of the prepuce that covers the neck and the bulb of the penis, and particularly the part that is related with the frenulum, is the most sensitive area of the penis.

CORPORA CAVERNOSA OF THE PENIS

The proximal three quarters of these two cylindrical masses of erectile tissue are closely joined and constitute the major portion of the penis body.

These corpora cavernosa separate at their base as they approach the pubic region. Each cylinder ends as a closed cone on the ventral face of the tuberosity of the ischium. The corpora cavernosa are firmly attached to it and to the pubis by the ischio cavernous muscle. The corpora cavernosa keeps its diameter unchanged until the distal end and terminates in a rounded form as it embeds itself on the glans or penis head.

The corpora cavernosa of the penis are surrounded by a strong fibrous cover that envelops both cylinders with its external fibers. Its internal fibers surround each cylinder separately, forming in the middle a septum that is incomplete in its most distal part. Each corpora cavernosa has a central artery and deep and surface dorsal veins. The structure of the corpora cavernosa is of the trabecular type rich in smooth muscles. These, as well as the arterial muscles, have the capacity of dilate and contract under the influence of the autonomous nervous system and of certain chemical substances that play a major role in the mechanism of erection.

The corpora spongiosa of the penis is the part that contains the urethra. It is also cylindrical but its diameter is smaller that of the corpora cavernosa. At its distal end, it expands to form the glans. Its posterior end also expands and forms the bulb of the penis, which connects with the bulbocavernous muscle.

The penile glans is the anterior end of the corpora spongiosa. It is conical in shape, its posterior diameter being larger than its anterior one, and its internal surface is connected with the corpora cavernosa. The part with the larger diameter constitutes the crown of the glans, next to which there is a constriction that forms an indentation on the neck of the penis. The participation of the corpora spongiosa in the mechanism of erection is minimal.

The prostate is a part glandular part muscular structure located right under the internal orifice of the urethra. It has the shape of a large walnut and it is situated in the pelvic cavity, under the symphysis of the pubis over the urogenital diaphragm and the rectum, which makes it possible to touch it through the rectum when it has enlarged.

The prostate is covered by a capsule consisting of fibrous tissue. Its muscular tissue constitutes its own stroma combined with trabecular shaped fibrous tissue. Its glandular part consists of epithelial cavities in the fibrous muscular network whose ducts end in the prostatic urethra. The bulbourethral glands (Cowpers glands) are two small round and lobular bodies located in the dorsal and lateral area of the membranous urethra close to the urethral bulb. Its secretion takes place in the cavernous segment of the urethra.

FEMALE GENITALIA

The female genitalia consist of an internal and an external group. The internal organs are located inside the pelvic cavity and include the ovaries, the uterine (or fallopian) tubes, the uterus, and the vagina. (Figs. 7, 8). The external organs include the mons pubis (or mons veneris), the labia majora, the labia minora, the clitoris, and the vestibular bulb. These components of the female genitalia, which are external to the urogenital diaphragm, are located under the pubic arc.

THE OVARIES

The ovaries are the counterpart of the male testicles. They are two nodular bodies located one on each side of the uterus with respect to the lateral wall of the pelvis. They are linked to the uterus by their broad ligament, dorsal and caudal in relation to the uterine tubes.

The ovary consists of a number of follicles encrusted in the mesh of connective tissue of the ovarian stroma. These follicles undergo a series of maturation changes culminating with ovulation. Under the influence of the hormones produced by the pituitary gland, there comes a moment when they break and expel a liquid and an ovule.

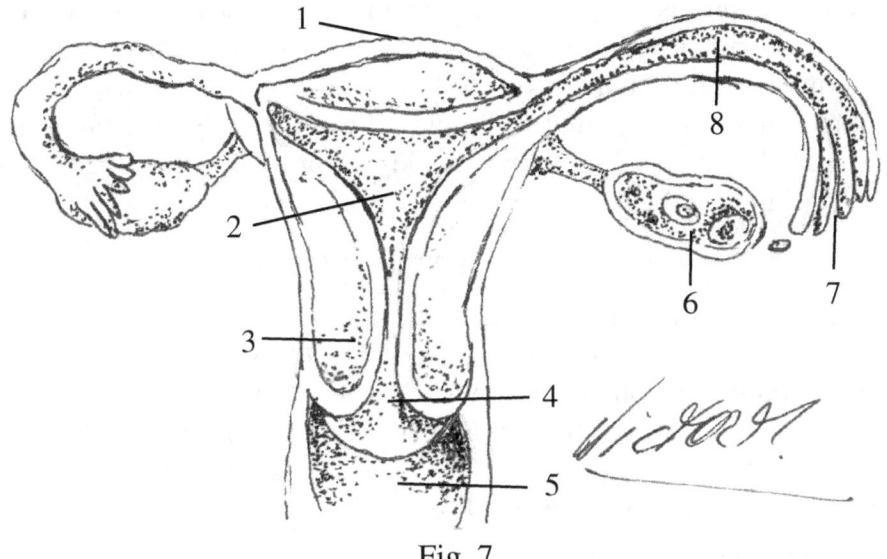

Fig. 7
Horizontal section of the internal female genital organs

1. Uterine fundus, 2. Uterine cavity, 3. Uterine neck, 4. Cervix,
5. Vagina, 6. Ovary, 7. Fimbria, 8. Fallopian tubes.

The liquid covers the peritoneal cavity and the ovule is deposited
on the fimbria of the uterine (or Fallopian) tube on the way to the
uterus, where it can be fertilized by the spermatozoa. This will happen
if the woman has had sex on the days before, during, or right after
ovulation.

After the follicle is ruptured, the corpus luteum is formed in its
cavity. If the ovule is fertilized the corpus luteum continues to grow
until the end of the ninth month. When the ovule is not fertilized,
a smaller corpus luteum is formed in the follicle that lasts until
menstruation and then atrophies.

THE UTERINE (OR FALLOPIAN) TUBES

The uterine tubes, one on each side, connect the ovary with the
uterus and transport the ovule towards the uterine cavity.

Their abdominal aperture is surrounded by an arboreal formation
called fimbriae that connect with the ovarian frimbriae. The other

extreme connects laterally with the uterine fundus and its cavity connects with the uterine cavity. The uterine tube consists of an external layer that continues in the peritoneum, a middle muscle layer composed of smooth muscle tissue laid out in a longitudinal and circular shape. An internal mucous layer connects with the mucous cover of the uterine cavity.

THE UTERUS

The uterus is a hollow, tubular and muscular organ located between the bladder and the rectum. It has the shape of a pear. The broad bottom section connects with the peritoneal cavity though the Fallopian tubes. The other extreme constitutes the uterine neck and extends into the vagina, which sticks to the uterus two centimeters from the extreme of the neck. The uterine cavity connects with the vagina through the cervical canal.

The connection of the uterus with the vagina forms a 90 degree angle. Its external layer comes from the peritoneum, which covers the whole intestinal surface and part of the surface related to the bladder. The middle layer, or myometrium, which constitutes most of the uterus, is part muscle and part blood and lymphatic vessels. The internal layer, or endometrium, consists of a mucous membrane whose cellular epithelium is characterized by tall columns of ciliary cells located in the body of the uterus. The internal layer of the uterus is very different from that of its neck. The mucous membrane covers the upper third of the neck cavity and consists of numerous deep glandular follicles that secrete a clear and viscous liquid with alkaline properties. The membrane covering the lower third of the canal shows numerous papillae whose epithelium becomes ciliary cells that gradually lose their cilia and get covered with a scaly stratified epithelium. On the vaginal side of the neck, the epithelium is also stratified and scaly, as in the vagina. During menstruation the uterus becomes enlarged and more vascular due to the fact that the mucous membrane gets thicker, softer and darker in color. These changes in the uterus are closely linked to the cyclic changes of the ovaries. The cycle is usually divided into four stages:

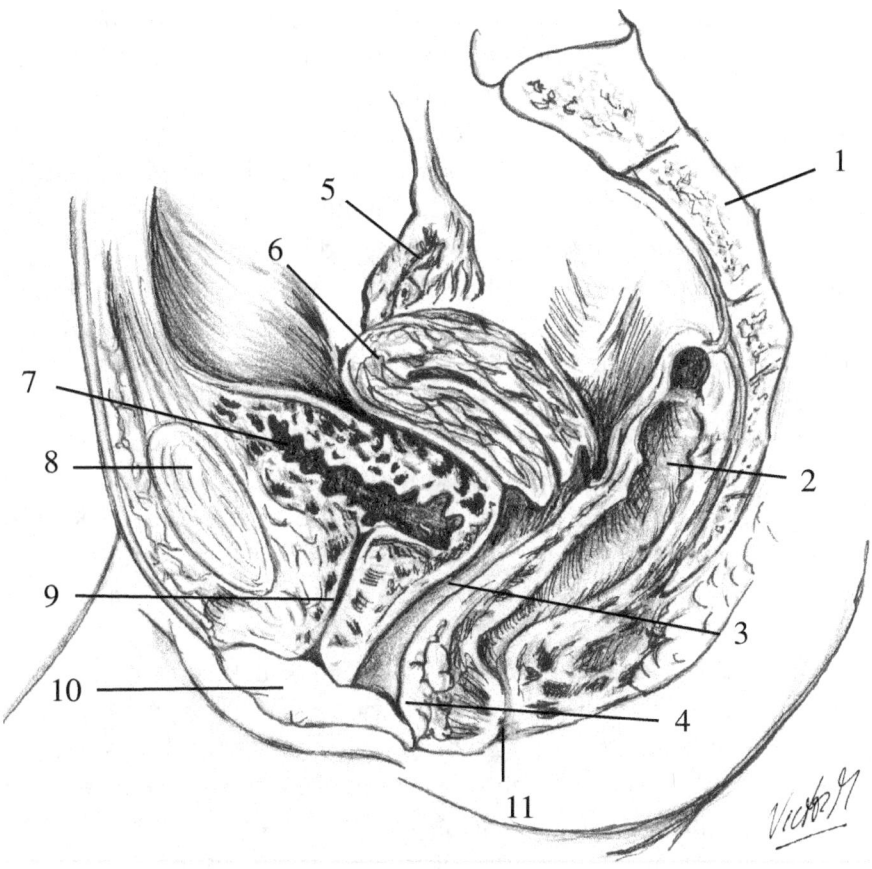

Fig. 8
Sagittal section of the female genital organs and rectum
1. Sacrum, 2. Rectum, 3. Vagina, 4. Bulb of vagina, 5. Ovary,
6. Uterus, 7. Bladder, 8. Pubis, 9. Urethra, 10. Labia mayora of
vulva, 11. Anus

1) Proliferative stage. The part of the endometrium adjacent to the
muscular layer, or myometrium, known as the basal layer, persists
until after menstruation, allowing the glands and the epithelium
to remain in an inactive state. After the menstrual flux is over, the
hormone responsible for follicular stimulation, produced by the

pituitary gland, triggers the growth of one of the ovarian follicles. As the follicle grows, it produces estrogen, a hormone that causes the proliferation of the endometrium and the growth of the uterine glands.

2) Secretory stage. When the ovarian follicle has matured to form what is called a Graaf follicle, it ruptures, often in the middle of the menstrual cycle, and discharges the ovule (or egg). Subsequently, under the influence of the pituitary gland, the follicle evolves to form the corpus luteum (or yellow corpus) whose cells multiply and produce the hormone called progesterone. This hormone stimulates and helps develop the glands in the endometrium. In addition, it lubricates and prepares the uterus to receive the fertilized egg.

3) Premenstrual stage. If the egg is fertilized it continues to grow. Otherwise, the corpus luteum starts to degenerate and stops the production of progesterone. At the same time the endometrium undergoes some changes in its vascularization, followed by deterioration of its tissue and fragmentation of its glands and epithelium.

4) Menstrual stage. The portion of the endometrium that contains enlarged glands and many blood capillaries is known as the functional epithelium or layer, to distinguish it from the basal glands and the tissue adjacent to the myometrium, known as the basal epithelium or layer. During menstrual discharge, the functional layer dies as a result of the rupture of blood vessels, which produces the hemorrhage associated with menstruation. The basal layer stays and reestablishes the endometrium for the next menstrual period.

THE VAGINA

The vagina extends from the vaginal vestibule to the uterus and is located between the bladder and the rectum. Its axis forms a 90 degree angle with the uterus. Its walls are in continuous contact. It is about 6 to 7.5 centimeters long on its ventral side and about 9 centimeters along its dorsal wall. It is narrow at the beginning, wider in the middle, and narrower at the uterine end, where it surrounds the vaginal segment of the uterine neck. The upper surface of the vagina is next to the bottom of the bladder and the urethra. Its back surface is separated from the rectum by the retrouterine hollow in its upper quarter, and by the recto-vaginal fascia in its two middle quarters. The lower quarter is separated from the anus and the rectum by perineal corpus.

The vagina consists of an internal mucous layer (mucous tunic) and a middle muscular layer, separated by a submucous layer of erectile tissue. The mucous tunic shows two longitudinal columns on its internal surface, one on the anterior wall and one on the posterior one. From these columns there arise a series of transversal formations that stand out giving the vaginal cavity its corrugated look. The tissue of the submucous layer is very elastic and it contains a plexus of large veins and soft muscle fibers intertwined, deriving from the muscle tunic.

The muscle tunic includes two layers. The external one, with its fibers oriented in a longitudinal manner, is the stronger layer, and its fibers continue as the surface muscle layers of the uterus. The strongest fascicles are attached to the rectovesicular fascia on both sides. On the internal muscle layer the muscle fibers are arranged in a circular fashion and its fascicles crisscross the longitudinal muscular fibers. In an area close to the entrance, the vagina is surrounded by an erectile tissue of the vestibule bulb and by strands of muscular fibers of the bulbocavernous muscle. The outermost layer of the vagina, consisting of connective tissue rich in blood vessels, overs the muscular tunic.

The external female genitalia consist of the mons pubis, the labia majora, the labia minora, the vestibular bulb, and the major vestibular glands. (Fig. 8)

The mons pubis is a round prominence located in the symphysis of the pubis. It consists of fatty tissue under the skin and it is covered by pubic hair after puberty.

The labia majora are two cutaneous formations or folds that extend laterally from the mons pubis to the perineum, forming a middle indenture.

The labia minora are two small cutaneous folds located between the labia majora. They extend laterally from the clitoris backwards in an oblique fashion for about 4 centimeters on each side of the vaginal orifice, terminating at the caudal area of the labia majora. In a virgin, the labia minora are joined at their distal or posterior end, forming a cutaneous fold or labial frenulum. Each of the labia minora is divided at its anterior end. The upper segment extends over the clitoris, covering the glans and forming the prepuce of the clitoris. The lower segment surrounds the clitoris from below and unites with the one from the opposite side to form the frenulum of the clitoris.

The clitoris is an erectile structure homologous to the penis. It is located behind the anterior labial fold and it is partially covered by the anterior edge of the labia minora. Its free end is a round prominence known as the glans of the clitoris. Like the penis, it has two corpora cavernosa consisting of erectile tissue surrounded by a fibrous layer. The posterior end of each corpus cavernosum is attached to the branches of the pubis and the isquium just like the penis. The clitoris also has a suspensory ligament and two small muscles on each side, the isquiocavernous muscles.

The aperture located between the labia minora and behind the glans of the clitoris is the vaginal vestibule. In it can be seen the orifice of the urethra and the entrance to the vaginal cavity.

The hymen is a thin fold of the mucous membrane located in the vaginal orifice. Its internal edge is normally in contact with the one from the opposite side outlining the entrance to the vagina. The hymen is highly variable in form. Most often it has the form of a ring but wider in the back. Sometimes it is a semilunar mucous fold with a concave edge on the side of the pubis. Occasionally it appears as a cribriform membrane. The hymen may also not be there, or it may show as a septum or wall along the lowest part of the vagina. This condition is known as unperforated hymen. Its presence should not be taken as a sign of virginity. The rupture of the hymen, associated with a minor hemorrhage during the first sexual act, depends primarily on the form and elasticity of the hymen. There may not be any hemorrhage during the first sexual act, so its value as a diagnostic of virginity is dubious.

The bulb of the vestibule consists of two masses of erectile tissue located at each side of the entrance of the vaginal wall and joined in their upper part by a band of tissue. In the back, the bulb expands and comes in contact with the major vestibular glands. Its inner surface is related with the surface layer of the urogenital diaphragm, and its outer layer is covered by the bulbocavernous muscle.

The major vestibular glands are homologous to the male bulbourethral glands. They consist of two small round masses located on each side of the entrance to the vagina. Each one is in contact with the back end of the bulbous mass of the vestibule. Each gland has a duct whose orifice faces the indentation formed by the hymen and the labia minora.

THE ANATOMIC BASIS OF THE SEXUAL ACT
NEUROPHYSIOLOGY

In order to understand the physiological changes that occur before, during, and after the sexual act, it is necessary to know the role played by the brain, the peripheral nerves that activate the sexual organs, and the arteries and veins that irrigate them. One must also take into account the important role played by male and female hormones and neurotransmitters.

The sexual function may look at first sight like sexual play. This is not so. From erection to ejaculation for the man, and excitation and orgasm for the woman, the sexual function is the result of the participation of many factors, including memories, caring, stimuli, hormonal and neural influences that originate in various parts of the brain and reach the genital organs through the spinal cord and the peripheral nervous system.

From a clinical point of view, the function of the brain may be analyzed on different levels.

The participation of the nervous system has been studied in part in relation to cerebral lesions of the areas that constitute the anatomical substratum of the sexual function. As for the brain stem, the reticular activating system of the mesencephalon (middle brain) and the pons, together with its conduits activated by dopamine, are responsible for maintaining an alert and vigilant state. When the activity of the reticular system decreases, the libido also diminishes or disappears. It must be remembered that any information that comes in and goes out does so through the brain stem towards or from the brain cortex, the limbic system, the spinal cord, the peripheral nerves, and the genital organs. A lesion to the brain stem may cause a change producing an inadequate information flow related to sexual activity and behavior.

Lesions to the nucleus of the tonsils in the hippocampus are associated with hypersexuality. Epileptic seizures due to traumatic lesions in the nucleus of the tonsils may exhaust dopamine as well as interfere with the secretion of the sexual hormones regulated by the hypothalamus-pituitary axis.

Stimulation of the hippocampus causes penile erection. It is believed that this neural structure has a modulating effect on the tumescence of the penis. Lesions to this area may interfere with erection.

Stimulation of the thalamus may also cause penile erection. Lesions to this area have been associated with hypersexual behavior.

The hypothalamus plays a very important role in the secretion of hormones and the sexual act. This organ integrates the information coming from the spinal cord, helps initiate and control the basic sexual response, and is associated with the sensation of sexual pleasure. Its cells secrete the hormone known as gonadotropin. This hormone, in turn, stimulates the release of the pituitary hormones that regulate functions like the menstrual cycle of women and the secretion of testosterone in men. Lesions to the hypothalamus may interfere with the production, secretion, and balance of hormones within the brain and the rest of the body. In children, lesions to the rear hypothalamus may cause a precocious puberty. In adults, this kind of lesion is associated with abnormalities like impotence in men and amenorrhea (lack of menstruation) in women. These disorders may be temporary or long-lasting.

The pellucid septum is associated with the sense of pleasure experienced right before and during orgasm. Damage to it may lead to impotence and loss of libido.

The pituitary gland and the hypothalamus work together as part of a complex system that regulates the production of various hormones in the human body. The anterior lobe of the pituitary gland reacts to the release of gonadotropin from the hypothalamus, which is then delivered to the pituitary gland through the blood vessels. The pituitary gland, in turn, secretes the gonadotropic hormones that stimulate the production of gonadic hormones by the ovaries, testicles, and other structures involved in reproduction and sexuality. In children, lesions to the pituitary gland are associated with lack or delay of puberty, or in some cases with precocious puberty. In adults it may cause sterility and lack of sexual drive. Lack of secretion is responsible for the decrease of secondary sexual characteristics.

Bilateral lesions to the temporal lobe and its connections with the tonsils may be associated with hypersexuality. More frequently, though, they produce epilepsy and a reduced sexual drive. Menstrual and reproductive disorders, weakening of the libido and sexual impotence are often seen in patients with epileptic seizures originating in the temporal lobe. Some of these patients may on occasion show unusual sexual behavior during the periods free of seizures, such as exhibitionism or fetishism.

The frontal lobe is related with the triggering and regulation of sexual activity and it helps modulate sexual behavior. Damage to the upper frontal or lateral dorsal areas often produces sexual apathy, lack of initiative and fantasy. Lesions to the orbital basal area lead to uninhibited and inappropriate sexual behavior.

The spinal cord, the peripheral somatic nerves, and the autonomous nervous system have a crucial role in the sexual act. The neural fibers that make up the autonomous nervous system deliver to the brain the external information of sexual stimulation, which is processed by various central neural structures. The brain then responds through neurotransmitters and activates the various organs involved in sexual activity during and after intercourse. Some of these impulses transmitted by the brain are conscious, but most of them are not.

The neural stimulation of male and female sexual organs is carried out by the somatic nerves originating in the sacral segments of the spinal cord, S2, S3, y S4, whose roots form the pudendal nerve. Its extremes activate the pelvic muscles, the sphincter, the skin neural terminals, the mucous membrane, the blood vessels, the penis, and the clitoris.

The autonomous or neurovegetative stimulation is carried out by the parasympathetic and the sympathetic nervous systems. The former originates in the sacral segment of the spinal cord, S2, S3 and

S4, giving origin to the splanchnic pelvic nerves. These are the motor and sensitive nerves of the bladder and its involuntary sphincter. Their stimulation triggers the act of urination. The arterial dilation produces erection of the penis and clitoris, tumescence of the vagina, and secretion of its glands, facilitating lubrication of the vulva and the vaginal cavity. In men, it produces lubrication through the action of its bulbourethral glands, as well as stimulating secretion by the prostate and the seminal vessels.

The sympathetic system originates in the lumbar area of the spinal cord, L1, L2 and L3. Its peripheral fibers form the hypogastric plexus and they activate the ureter muscle, the trigonal muscle, and the muscle of the urethral crest. It also activates the muscles of the epididymis, the vas deferens, the seminal vesicle, and the prostate. Stimulation of the hypogastric plexus produces ejaculation of the seminal fluid into the urethra. The sympathetic system has a constricting effect on the blood vessels and the soft muscles of the corpora cavernosa of the penis, the clitoris and the vascular layer of the vagina. Its action coincides with orgasm and leads to the resolution of the sexual act.

Sex Hormones

Sexual behavior is a physiological function, as it depends in great part on the morphology of the genital organs and the male and female hormones. The sexual drive is controlled by the hormones particular to each sex. Thus, a castrated man will lose all interest in sexual activity due to the absence of the hormones that control that type of behavior. The sex hormones have a distinct role in sexual activity, manifested by their effect on the organization of the sexual organs and the psychosexual orientation of the brain. Male and female brains are different due to the influence of their distinct hormones. We could say the brain has a specific gender.

It is a known fact that men and women react differently to the situations they face. Men tend to be promiscuous and aggressive, while women are faithful and affectionate. It is no wonder, then, that many of the behavior patterns of men and women are different, since the brain is functionally different, with substantial variation in the hypothalamus and the cortex due to hormonal influence, androgenous for men, and estrogenous for women.

In order for hormones to have an effect on the organization of a person's character, they must act at an early stage in the development of the brain. In humans, this takes place in the fetus. Most of the relevant studies have been conducted in laboratory rats. The most noticeable changes have been observed in the effect of testosterone on the formation of synaptic connections between the neural cells of the hypothalamus and the pre-optical area in adult rats.

These morphological differences between the male and the female brain have given rise to much speculation on the mathematical capacity of men and intuition in women. What matters most is that these structural differences in the brain are reflected primarily in sexual activity, procreation, care of children, and affective relations.

Maternal behavior is determined by these neural and hormonal mechanisms that lead to the establishment of an affective relationship between mother and child. The suction reflex, crying, smiling, and later hugging and verbal communication, guarantee the creation of an emotional tie between mother and child.

These experimental results and the observation of maternal behavior point to the important influence that hormones have on the brain with respect to loving relationships. In addition to these physiological factors, we must no doubt take into account other factors that affect an individual's development, such as the social family environment.

In men as well as in women there exist hormones that are essential for the development and continuation of sexuality. We will describe them separately.

TESTOSTERONE

A man's testicles secrete various sexual hormones, collectively known as androgenous, including testosterone, dihydrotestosterone, and androstenedione. The most abundant and important of these is testosterone. This hormone is converted to a more active form, the dihydrosterone, which is present in the prostate and in the external genital organs of the male fetus.

Testosterone is secreted by the so-called Leydig interstitial cells, located between the seminipherous tubes of the testicles. These cells are almost non-existent in children but are very abundant in newly born boys and in adults after puberty. In both of these stages they secrete a large amount of testosterone.

Androgenous hormones are also produced in tissues other than the testicles. The supra-renal glands secrete at least five different types of androgenous hormones. Their influence in the development of male characteristics is minimal and they do not produce any male characteristics in women, except pubic and axillary hair.

The function of testosterone, in general, is the development of male sexual characteristics, including the formation of the penis, the scrotum, the prostatic gland, seminal vesicles, and genital ducts, during the fetal stage.

During puberty, secretion of testosterone is reactivated, causing the growth of the penis, the scrotum, and the testicles, which are the primary male sexual traits. Testosterone is also responsible for the development of secondary characteristics that start with puberty and end with maturity. Secondary sexual characteristics, just like the genital organs themselves, are different in men and in women. Testosterone causes the growth and distribution of pubic hair, as well as hair around the belly button or higher, facial hair, and hair around the thorax or, less frequently, in other parts of the body. It also contributes to slowing down the growth of hair on top of the head. Disregarding genetic factors, it is said that a man that does not have a normal testicular function never becomes bald.

Changes of the voice in puberty are due to the fact that testosterone produces hypertrophia of the mucous membrane and growth of the larynx, gradually leading to a typical masculine voice. The skin also undergoes changes due to hormonal influence. It gets rougher and the subcutaneous tissue becomes thicker. The muscular system also shows noticeable changes, due to the formation of muscular protein and other types of protein that are deposited in different parts of the body.

Due to the great influence of testosterone on muscular structure, it is often used by athletes to improve muscular strength. Sometimes they use synthetic androgenous hormones instead. This is a very dangerous practice, since an excess of testosterone may produce hirsuteness (too much hair), priapism (constant erection), polycythemia (excessive number of red cells in the blood), high cholesterol, and brain vessel malfunctions, among other things. Neither is it justified for old people to use testosterone as a "youth hormone".

Another effect of testosterone is the growth of bones and an increase in calcium deposits. Finally, testosterone has a specific effect in the configuration of the male pelvis.

Under the influence of the gonadotropin hormones produced by the pituitary gland, the testicles maintain the capacity to produce sperm from puberty through the rest of a man's life. Most men, however, start to show a slow decrease in their sexual drive around the age of 50. One study showed that the median age of termination of sexual activity is 68, but there is considerable variation. The decrease of sexual desire is related to the decrease in the secretion of testosterone. The weakening of the sexual drive in men is know as the male climacteric, which is occasionally accompanied by shortness of breath, hot flashes, and psychic disorders similar to those experienced by women during menopause. These symptoms may be corrected by administering testosterone or some synthetic androgenous hormone.

ESTROGEN

The main function of estrogen is the proliferation and development of the female sexual organs and other tissues involved in reproduction. During childhood, estrogen is secreted in minimal amounts, but this changes with puberty, when its production, thanks to the pituitary gland, may increase twenty times or more. During this stage, the female sexual organs acquire the characteristics they will have in adulthood. The ovaries, the Fallopian tubes, the uterus, and the vagina become larger. So do the external genital organs: the mons veneris (due to fat deposits), the labia majora, and the labia minora.

During the years that follow puberty, estrogen changes the vaginal type of epithelium, which becomes stratified and consequently more resistant to trauma and infection. The uterus also keeps growing, and its endometrial epithelium is later used to help feed the implanted ovule. In the Fallopian tubes, the mucous epithelium also changes. It proliferates and becomes ciliated, which favors the propulsion of the fertilized egg towards the uterus. The breasts undergo big changes: their tissue grows, there are more fat deposits, and a system of ducts is developed. There are also changes produced by two other hormones, progesterone and prolactin, which complete the development of the breasts and convert them into milk producing organs.

Estrogen has a strong effect on the growth of the skeleton, leading to the early union of the epiphysis with the axis of the long bones.

Deficiency of estrogen after menopause produces osteoporosis. Fat deposits on the subcutaneous tissue, due to estrogen, appear mainly on the hips and the thighs, producing the typical female body.

Estrogen does not have a significant effect of the distribution of hair. It is mainly the androgenous hormones produced by the supra-renal glands that are responsible for pubic and axillary hair.

PROGESTERONE

This hormone originates in the corpus luteum of the ovaries, under the influence of the pituitary gland. Its main function is to trigger the secretional changes of the uterine endometrium during the second half of the female menstrual cycle to prepare the uterus for the implantation of a fertilized egg. It also helps decrease the frequency of uterine contractions to prevent the expulsion of the egg once it has been implanted. The epithelium of the uterus increases its secretion for the nourishment of the egg as it moves toward the uterus. It also triggers the development of lobes and alveoli in the breasts and it facilitates the proliferation of alveolar cells, converting them into secretional glands. The increase in size of the breasts is also due to fluid retention in the subcutaneous tissue. The endometrial and menstrual cycles are described in general terms in the section on anatomy and physiology.

Between the ages of 40 and 50 the menstrual cycle becomes irregular and ovulation loses the regularity it had before. This phenomenon, characterized by a decrease in sexual hormones and cessation of the cycles, is known as menopause. During this stage, women must readjust their lives, which so far have been stimulated by the production of estrogen and progesterone. The lack of estrogen often causes noticeable physiological changes, including hot flashes, shortness of breath, irritability, fatigue, anxiety, and in some cases psychotic outbursts. These symptoms are serious in about 15 per cent of women, and they require treatment with small daily doses of estrogen, progressively reduced, in order to prevent the continuation of the symptoms.

PROLACTIN

Estrogen and progesterone are essential for the development of the breasts during pregnancy. A specific effect of these hormones is the inhibition of milk production. Prolactin has exactly the opposite effect, that is, it stimulates milk production. Its importance in sexuality is related to hypersecretion controlled by the hypothalamus. What is interesting is that under normal conditions the hypothalamus stimulates the production of all hormones but it inhibits the production of prolactin. For this reason, lesions of the hypothalamus are associated with an increase in the production of prolactin. Tumors in the pituitary gland, as well as some medications, may cause hypersecretion of prolactin. A high level of prolactin in the blood produces galactorrhea and inhibition of sexual desire, both in men and women.

Physiology of Intercourse

The physiological effects of intercourse have been studied in the laboratory under artificial circumstances with the participation of young couples. The data obtained from these studies suggest that sexual activity is associated with noticeable fluctuations of the cardiovascular system, including acceleration of the heartbeat from 110 to 180 beats per minute, and significant increase of blood pressure from 40 to 80 mm. at the contraction stage. Breath rate also increases, from 30 to 60 breaths per minute. Although these changes are dramatic, their duration is short, reaching their peak right before or during orgasm, and returning to their normal values after a few minutes. It is important to keep these changes in mind when dealing with patients that have cardiovascular deficiencies.

THE MALE SEXUAL ACT

The most important source of impulses leading to the sexual act is the penis. Besides the crown of the glans, the area right behind it and the ventral section of the penis (with respect to the frenulum) contain sensitive neural terminals that transmit to the central system the special modality of sensation known as a sexual sensation. Digital massage, labial and lingual caresses of other parts of the body, such as the neck, ears, abdomen, scrotum, groin, nipples, although they do not involve strictly sexual areas, produce a pleasing sensation that increases and integrates with the sexual sensation when it is produced at the right moment. This type of stimulation, produced before the introduction of the penis in the vagina, is known as foreplay, and it is very important for the woman. Foreplay allows the woman to get ready for intercourse, through the activation of the major verstibular glands (Bartholin's glands) that secrete a fluid that lubricates the labia majora, the labia minora, and the entrance to the vagina. Once the vagina is lubricated, penile penetration produces friction of the glans against the vaginal wall, which leads to the sexual sensation due to stimulation of its neural terminals transmitted by the pudendum nerve and the sacral plexus to the sacral area of the spinal cord. In addition, the impulses originating from areas adjacent to the penis also contribute to sexual stimulation. Once those stimuli have reached the spinal cord they make their way to different areas of the brain. Sexual sensations may even originate in other internal structures, like the urethra, the bladder, the prostate, the seminal vesicles, the testicles, and the vas deferens. The stimulation of these organs is associated with sexual secretions and impulses that may in some cases be constant. Appropriate psychological stimuli increase a person's ability to perform the sexual act. Thought and fantasies with sexual content, or even dreaming of having sex, may result in erection and ejaculation. Nocturnal emissions during an erotic dream occur frequently in men during puberty.

Psychological factors often play an important role in the sexual act. They may either trigger or inhibit it. It is possible that the brain is not necessary for its realization, since an adequate genital stimulation may produce ejaculation in animals, and occasionally in men whose spinal cord has been cut in the lumbar area. This suggests that the sexual act may respond to reflexes of the sacral and lumbar areas of the spine. These reflexes may be triggered by a physical or a psychological stimulus, but most likely by a combination of the two.

PHASES OF THE MALE SEXUAL ACT

ERECTION

Erection is the first effect of sexual stimulation in men. The degree of erection is proportional to the degree of psychological and physical stimulation. Erection is important in stimulating active participation by the woman. Unfortunately, women are generally passive at the beginning of the sexual act. This derives from ignorance and the idea that if a woman takes the initiative, her behavior will be interpreted as that of a prostitute. This idea is completely erroneous, since a prostitute is only interested in getting her customer to have an orgasm as soon as possible, and does not have the affectionate attitude that exists in a couple whose interpersonal relation is richer in every sense. The prostitute "has sex", while the couple joined by affection "makes love". At the initial stage of the sexual act, it is important for both men and women to engage in foreplay. This consists, as explained before, of caresses involving tactile and oral stimulation of certain parts of the body including the genitals. Participation in foreplay must be mutual, spontaneous, uninhibited, and delicate, without causing pain or discomfort. This physical aspect is complemented by the psychological stimulation provided by pleasant past experiences and fantasies. Foreplay must be varied and not always follow the same routine, unless the couple enjoys the same type of stimulation and does not get bored. What matters is that every time the couple wants to make love, both partners should have the right emotional disposition to participate and share in the erotic pleasure of foreplay and intercourse.

The stimulus thus initiated results in erection due to the autonomous parasympathetic system. The impulses originating in the brain or the sacral spinal cord reach the penis through the erectile nerves. These parasympathetic impulses dilate the penile arteries and relax the soft muscles of the corpora cavernosa and spongiosa that are covered with a firm fibrous membrane. This facilitates the blood flow and an increase of pressure in the erectile tissue, which resembles a sponge consisting of venous sinusoids and a cavernous structure. These are normally almost empty, but they expand considerably during stimulation. Due to the increase in arterial flow and pressure in the corpora cavernosa, the venous outflow diminishes resulting in partial blocking. Since both corpora cavernosa are surrounded by a strong fibrous membrane, the blood flow and high pressure inside them produces an increase in diameter, elongation and hardening of the penis.

LUBRICATION

During sexual stimulation, the parasympathetic system, in addition to triggering erection, stimulates the urethral and bulbo-urethral glands, producing a mucous secretion that exits through the urethra and facilitates lubrication during intercourse. However, the greater part of lubrication is provided by the glands of the female sexual organs. Without appropriate lubrication the sexual act is unpleasant and irritating. It may produce pain and inhibition of sexual sensations.

EMISSION AND EJACULATION

These two phases are a function of the autonomous vegetative sympathetic system. They are the culminating moment of the male sexual act. When the sexual stimulus increases, the reflex centers of the spinal cord start emitting sympathetic impulses that exit at the lumbar area and reach the genital organs though the hypogastric and pelvic plexus to initiate emission and culminate in ejaculation. Emission starts with the contraction of the deferens ducts leading to expulsion of the sperm in the urethra. This leads immediately to contraction of the muscular layer of the prostate and the seminal vesicles and consequent ejection of prostatic and seminal fluids that pushes the sperm forward. The mixture of these fluids in the urethra with the ones secreted by the bulbo-urethral glands constitutes what we call semen. This phase of the process is known as emission.

The contents of the urethra produces sensations that are transmitted by the pudendal nerves to the sacral area of the spinal cord and are perceived as rapid fullness of the internal genital organs. These sensations, in turn, produce rhythmic contractions of the muscular layer of the internal genital organs and the ischio cavernous and bulbo-cavernous muscles that compress the erectile tissue at the base of the penis. This causes an increase in pressure inside the genital ducts and the urethra in the form of rhythmic waves leading to the expulsion of the semen from the urethra. This process is known as ejaculation. At the same time, the intense rhythmic contractions of the pelvic muscles and the trunk intensify the movement of the pelvis facilitating penetration by the penis. This contributes to the expulsion of the semen in the deepest part of the vagina and even at the entrance to the neck of the uterus. The period of emission and ejaculation constitutes the male orgasm.

Pleasure reaches its climax at the moment of ejaculation. It becomes more intense if it coincides with muscular contraction of the woman's perineum and rhythmic movement of her hips. The sensation of pleasure ends with a slightly painful sensation around the glans of the penis that prevents further rhythmic movement and leads to withdrawal of the penis from the vagina. During this short pleasure phase, there are rapid respiratory and cardiovascular changes that give way to a state of normalcy in a few minutes. This phase, followed by a state of relaxation probably related to the production of endorphins, is known as resolution. It is characterized by a sensation of muscular relaxation and general calm that may produce sleepiness. The penis returns to its flaccid state, although with young men it may remain in a state of tumescense.

Erotic pleasure is intense, special, and unique, due to the sensation itself and the physiological changes that go with it. Mutual pleasure as a physical sensation and emotional satisfaction experienced when there is true sharing is very important for the long-term coexistence of the couple.

THE FEMALE SEXUAL ACT

For the woman the success of the sexual act depends not only on psychological and physical stimulation but also on a satisfactory emotional relation with her partner. For her, participation in the sexual act has a more complex emotional significance than for the man. The woman gives herself to the man as an expression of love and the desire to satisfy him. The sexual relation of a couple united by the desire to coexist will provide, through a harmonious interpersonal relation, the pattern for the woman to be emotionally disposed to share the erotic experience. We must emphasize the importance of education, her knowledge of her own body, and the myths and taboos that have been a part of her sexual development. Taking this into account and assuming that these factors have not produced a negative disposition toward sexuality, the physiological description of the female sexual act will not differ significantly from that of the male sexual act.

PHASES OF THE FEMALE SEXUAL ACT

STIMULATION

The first phase is sexual stimulation. The success of the sexual act depends on a well balanced stimulation both psychologically and physically. Erotic thoughts and fantasies help awaken sexual desire in women. Quite possibly this desire is partially based on the woman's predisposition and partially on physiological impulses and the production of the right kind of hormones. Sexual desire varies according to the menstrual cycle, reaching its maximum at the time of ovulation, due to the high level of estrogens during the pre-ovulation period, that is, the days around the middle of the menstrual cycle. Sexual stimulation in women is similar to that in men. Particularly important is tactile or oral stimulation of the clitoris. Tactile stimulation of the vulva, vagina or other areas of the perineum may also trigger sexual desire. Irritation of these organs or of the urinary tract may also trigger sexual sensations. Just like in men, these sensations are transmitted to the sacral area of the spinal cord through the pudedum nerve and the sacral plexus. Once they enter the spinal cord they are transmitted to the brain. Female sexual desire is also influenced by reflex integration in the lumbar and sacral areas of the spinal cord.

Stimulation of nonsexual organs is also important for awakening sexual desire in women as part of foreplay. The ears, the neck, the breasts, the abdomen, the back, the groin, the inside of the thighs, are erogenous zones that when tenderly caressed with the hands or the lips will predispose the woman to engage herself in the erotic experience. The stimulus will be more effective if the interpersonal relation has been satisfactory as far as communicating emotional needs and satisfaction and the desire to share and mutually enjoy every moment in harmonious coexistence. Given these conditions, the woman will feel free to express her satisfaction and feel wanted. With her female intuition she will be able to provide more variety to foreplay, since her capacity for erotic imagination is greater than the man's. Rough and tactless stimulation will have a negative effect, as it will inhibit sexual desire and affection.

ERECTION AND LUBRICATION

Erectile tissue in women is located at the entrance to the vagina and in the clitoris. This erectile tissue is almost identical to that of men. It is under the control of the parasympathetic nerves that cross the erectile nerves from the sacral plexus to the external genital organs. At the early stage of sexual stimulation, the parasympathetic impulses dilate the arteries of the erectile tissue located at the entrance to the vagina. This allows the vagina wall to become congested, thus facilitating greater contact with the penis and triggering a sufficient sexual stimulus to make ejaculation possible. The parasympathetic impulses activate Bartholin's glands, which are located behind the labia minora, and make them secrete a mucous fluid into the entrance to the vagina. This mucus is in great part responsible for lubrication during intercourse. The vagina is also lubricated by fluid from the male urethral glands. Appropriate lubrication of the vagina is essential so that friction with the penis will produce a pleasant sensation culminating with a climax for both the man and the woman.

Foreplay prior to penile penetration is very important, as it allows for adequate stimulation of the woman as well as lubrication of the vaginal duct. If vaginal lubrication is inadequate, penetration of the penis produces an irritating, unpleasant, and painful sensation in the woman.

ORGASM

The general perception of the frequency with which women attain orgasm is incorrect. The studies on sexuality published by Kinsey in 1945 indicated that married women as a group experience orgasm only in 30 percent of the cases, where orgasm is understood as genital to genital stimulation. Not included in these studies are cases of orgasm produced by tactile or oral stimulation of the female genitalia. According to a more recent study of 100 married couples between the ages of 30 and 40 who consider themselves happy, the frequency of orgasm for the woman is only 46 percent.

For a long time, female orgasm was not considered a mark of success, and men had the idea that such an erotic and pleasing sensation did not exist. It was only with the advent of Freud that sex started to be discussed in public and the idea of female orgasm became more widely accepted.

The general consensus was that true orgasm was only produced through vaginal stimulation by the penis. This implied that any orgasm produced by a different kind of stimulation was unhealthy or even immoral, sinful and corrupt. This idea has been devastated for the many women who were unable to experience orgasm through vaginal stimulation. Later studies confirmed that most women can only attain orgasm through direct stimulation of the clitoris, which is a rudimentary form of the male penis. Fortunately, this way of obtaining sexual pleasure is now considered normal. The area that is sensitive to stimulation by the penis is located in the anterior and superior third of the vagina, probably in relation with the urethra. It has been designated the "G spot" in honor of the German gynecologist Dr. Ernest Grafenberg, who described it in 1950, although he did not present histological evidence. From an anatomical point of view, we must keep in mind that the labia majora , the labia minora, the outer third of the vaginal canal, the vulva, and the vulvar vestibule are all very rich in neural structure. Another anatomical component of this area are the bulbo-cavernous muscles, whose voluntary contraction produces a narrowing of the entrance to the vagina, thus contributing to greater friction of the penis with the vaginal cavity. This increase in friction stimulates both the neural terminals of the penis and the outer third of the vagina. If a woman knows something about her genital anatomy, she can control the contraction of those muscles and increase the sexual sensation during penetration by the penis.

An important factor for women who attain a good muscle tone during intercourse is the use of a lubricating cream, such as vaseline, which contains a pure petroleum jelly. It has the advantage of adhering to the skin and the mucous membrane without totally disappearing with the secretions of the penis and the vulva. This cream must be applied both to the glans and body of the penis and to the entrance of the vulva.

The sexual sensation of pleasure originates in this segment of the vagina, due to friction by the penis. As this sensation increases, rhythmic contractions of the outer third of the vaginal canal start, as well as rhythmic contractions of the uterus, which intensify as the pleasure becomes more intense. At the same time, the muscles of the perineum, the abdomen and even the face undergo intense contraction, voluntary or subconscious, in association with intense pleasure. Women explain that vaginal pleasure originates in the upper wall of the superior and anterior third of the vagina, later extending to the deep area of the perineum and ending with a sensation of pleasure in the lumbar area. This sensation is, like in men, unique in character and intensity, and lasts no more than 30 or 40 seconds. The reaction of the organism is total.

The anterior and superior third of the vagina is adequately stimulated by penile penetration in certain positions. One of them is with the woman lying on her back and her pelvis raised by a pillow. Raising of the pelvis may also be done by the woman flexing and elevating her legs, or by the man placing his hands under the woman's hips and raising them at the moment of penetration. Some women prefer to take a more active role in intercourse, with the man lying on his back and the woman sitting on top of him, thus controlling vaginal penetration and the antero-posterior movement of the pelvis.

A slight variant of this position is with the woman turning her back towards the man and placing her knees at each side of his pelvis so as to control vaginal penetration. While the woman performs the antero-posterior movement, the man matches her rhythm elevating his pelvis so as to facilitate penetration and contact of the penis with the upper anterior part of the vagina. Another alternative is for the woman to lie on her side with one or both legs flexed over her abdomen, and for the man to penetrate her from behind. This facilitates contact of the glans with the most sensitive area of the vagina, but is problematic if the woman is obese or the man's penis is small. In another variant the man sits on a chair and the woman straddles him, controlling penetration and the antero-posterior rhythmic movements of her hips. The existence of an erogenous zone in the vagina and the sensibility of the clitoris constitute the neurophysiological basis of sexual stimulation and orgasm for the woman. However, the attainment of erotic pleasure for a couple implies additional factors that we will now analyze. One of them is a normal physical development with its hormonal component. Hormonal deficiencies and genital anomalies play an important role in the awakening of erotic sensations and the performance of the sexual act.

Another important factor is education, particularly as it concerns knowledge of human sexuality. Unfortunately, neither men nor women are exposed to formal instruction in this area. Most of the information gathered by young men and women prior to sexual experience is obtained "on the street", and lacks any of the basic facts of anatomy, neurophysiology and psychology. What is transmitted from generation to generation is mainly myths and taboos. Sex education ought to be an essential part of the curriculum. What young people usually get in school are only some notions of the physiology of procreation, menstruation, and the risk of venereal diseases. There are several factors that conspire against an integral sexual education of young people: parents' lack of information, absence of responsible people with sexual experience, and restrictions imposed by religion or pseudo-morality. What young people get is partial and incomplete, and cannot lead to the development and practice of normal sexuality.

The conception of sexuality that exists in most homes is often erroneous. There is a predominance of negative ideas and attitudes that can only lead to mistaken concepts and confusion regarding psycho-sexual matters in the minds of young people. Talk of indignity, evil, sin, degeneration, and filth is what most 4 or 5 year old children hear when they begin manifesting sexual curiosity and exploration. Clinical experience shows an abundance of psychological trauma dating back to this early age that prevents men and women from developing a normal erotic experience.

Sexual relations without adequate information may produce a satisfactory orgasmic experience but they are not a proper foundation for a long-term sustained relationship. In this case sexual satisfaction may be affected by various factors. If communication is not spontaneous, unconditional, open, and honest, people's expression of desires, inclinations, likes and dislikes, what pleases and what frustrates, may cause misunderstanding and confrontation.

One's personal ability to express feelings of caring, love, and friendship projected towards another person will facilitate the free sharing of what one thinks and feels. If an individual involved in a long term relationship lacks the ability to communicate or share affection, emotions, and common interests, the couple may easily end up in a routine existence that in the long run will lead to the acceptance of an interaction without any personal involvement. Boredom, anxiety, depression, and the fake reality of being together yet feeling lonely may gradually erode mutual communication. Add to this one's own frustrations and problems, and the situation becomes more intolerable. The pleasure of a true erotic experience is much broader than just sexual satisfaction.

Just as in men, female orgasm is accompanied by heightened blood pressure, reaching its maximum at the moment of climax and returning to its normal values afterwards. There is also accelerated breath that may cause hyperventilation and even apnea in some cases.

RESOLUTION OR RELAXATION PHASE

The next state is one of resolution or relaxation mediated, just as in men, by the production of endorphins. This phase is slower in women than in men. With practice, some women may have two or more orgasms. This is why women are said to be multiorgasmic.

Following orgasm, the erection of the nipples decreases and the congestion of the skin and the vagina returns to its normal state. Due to the relaxation of the vagina after orgasm, the neck of the uterus descends towards the sperm deposited by the semen. After reaching the climax, women's temperature, blood pressure, and pulse return to their normal values, just as they do in men.

The general sensation of relaxation may lead to a state of sleepiness, which may not be appreciated if it affects only one member of the couple.

Vaginal Penetration Positions

The number of positions during intercourse is highly variable. Textbooks describe a great variety of them. Some of them are more effective than others in stimulating the vagina, which is the most important consideration. Others are simply devised to produce erotic excitement for the man. Thus, depending on the physical and athletic condition of the man, there are numerous positions for vaginal penetration. We will describe only the basic ones that are most effective for vaginal stimulation. Couples should feel free to experiment with any position that produces mutual satisfaction.

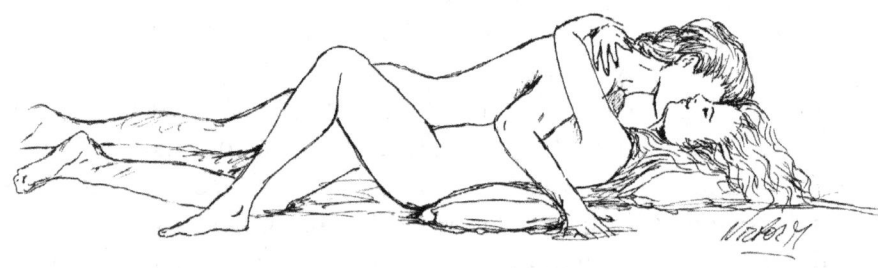

Position 1 (Fig. 9)

The woman lies on her back with her legs bent at the knees and her hips raised by a pillow or cushion.

In this positon, perhaps the most common, the woman rests on her back with her legs separated and extended or somewhat flexed. The man lies on top between the woman's legs. In spite of being the most common position, it is the least stimulating for the woman since it does not lead to adequate friction of the penis against the upper external third of the vagina. This is the most sensitive area where the bulbocavernous muscles are located, which the woman may contract during penetration so as to increase friction. This may be one of the most pleasant positions for both partners if a pillow is placed under the woman's hips or if the man raises them with his hands. The woman's legs must be semi-flexed. By raising the pelvis, the penis penetrates the vagina in an oblique fashion and is able to stimulate the sensitive area previously mentioned.

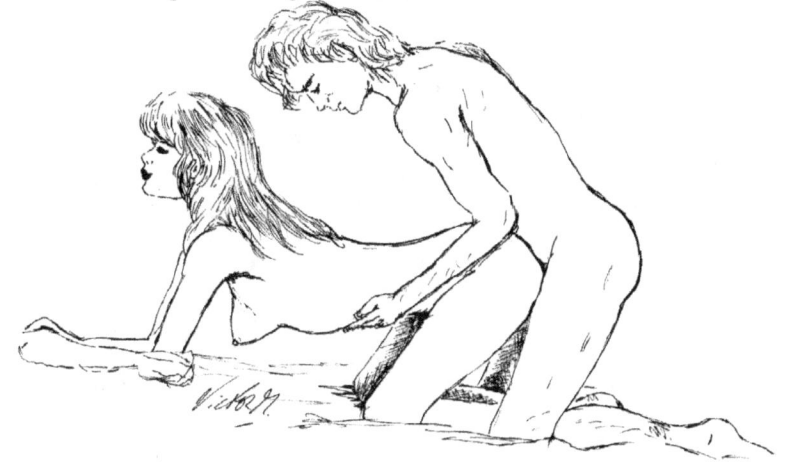

Position 2 (Fig. 10)
Both the man and the woman on their knees.

The woman is on her knees and supports herself with her elbows or hands. She can also kneel on the floor with her body resting on the bed. Vaginal penetration is from behind. In one of the variants, both partners lie on their sides, the man behind the woman. If the man rests on his left side, his left leg is extended and makes contact with the woman's left leg, also extended. To achieve penetration, the man's right leg crosses the woman's left leg and makes contact with the back of the woman's right leg which is semi-flexed.

After penetration both partners may flex their legs keeping good contact and maintaining penetration from behind. This position in any of its variants is not recommended if the woman is obese or the man's penis is small.

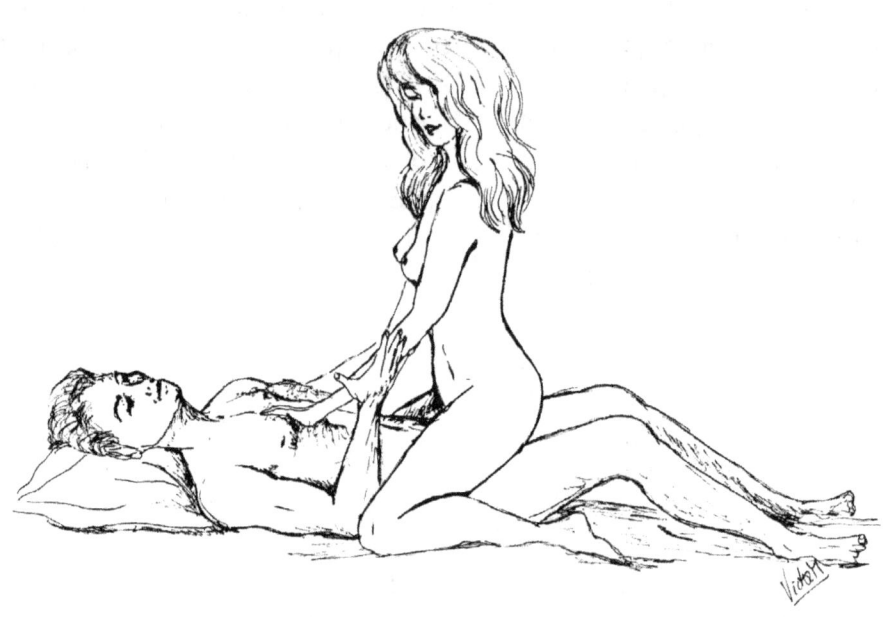

Position 3 (Fig. 11)

The man lies on his back. The woman sits on top of him with her knees flexed.

The man rests on his back. The woman sits on top of him facing him. Vaginal penetration is from the front. The woman controls penetration with the back and forward motion of her pelvis. This is one of the most satisfactory positions for the woman, allowing her to reach a climax through adequate stimulation of the upper wall of the external third of the vagina.

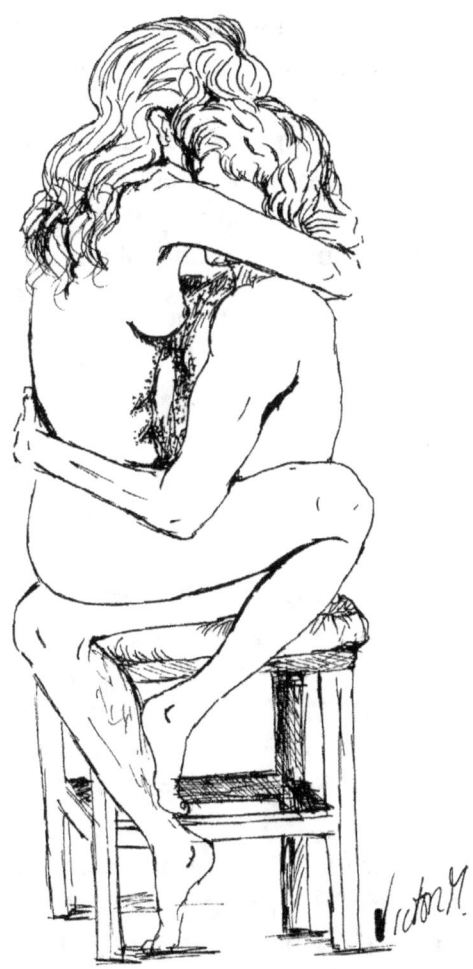

Position 4 (Fig. 12)
The man sits on a chair or bench, and the woman sits on his thighs
facing him.

The man is sitting on a chair or bench, and the woman straddles him. This position also allows the woman to have control of penetration and movement of her pelvis. The man may either be passive or lift his hips at the time of penetration. The sitting position helps prevent premature ejaculation. The woman stops moving as soon as the man signals the beginning of a sensation of pleasure. Once this dissipates, the woman starts the cycle again. She may do this up to ten times, and then allow him to ejaculate.

In another variant, the woman faces away from the man, and penetration is from behind. She controls penetration and the movement of her hips. The position may vary. The woman may lean back or rest her back against the man's abdomen. On this variant the man controls penetration and can stimulate the clitoris with his middle finger.

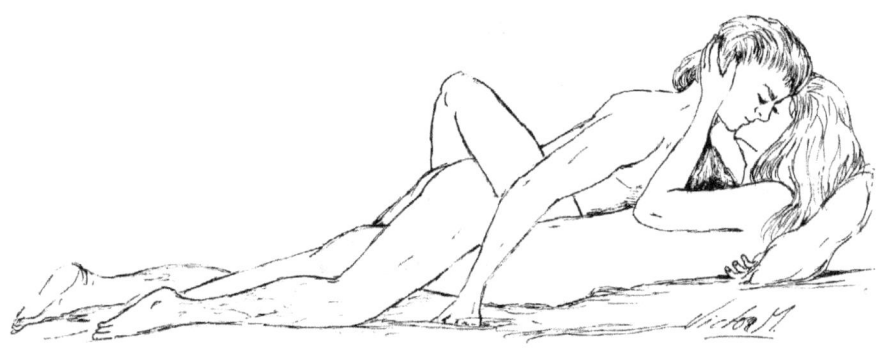

Position 5 (Fig. 13)

On this position the woman lies on her back and the man lies on his side to the right side of the woman, who bends her right leg. The man's right leg crosses the woman's left leg, and the man penetrates the vagina while lying on his side. This allows him to stimulate the clitoris with his right middle finger. When the woman starts to feel pleasure, the man gets on top of her while she keeps her right leg bent, as shown on figure 13. This is a comfortable position for men suffering from lumbar problems. The woman has the opportunity of reaching orgasm through stimulation of both the clitoris and the vagina. Vaginal stimulation is achieved through penetration of the penis

If any of these positions make it possible to have an orgasm, it must be kept in mind that a harmonious relation and the practice of foreplay prior to intercourse are very important to help the woman be sexually satisfied.

It is also important to emphasize that during intercourse the man should always have a positive attitude towards his partner, acting with tenderness and caring so that the woman receives the message of affection that she needs and expects from the man she loves.

Patients with heart problems or other physical handicaps should try to find the most appropriate position that will allow them not to exert themselves too much.

If the lubrication produced by foreplay is not sufficient, it is advisable to use a cream so that the friction of the penis on the vagina does not cause irritation.

Orgasm

DETERMINING FACTORS

The desired outcome of intercourse is the attainment of orgasm or sexual climax, characterized by the sensation of pleasure described previously. It constitutes the goal of the couple engaged in the sexual act.

For men it is rare not to have an orgasm during the sexual act. Generally they need a short period of foreplay to get excited enough to engage in sexual intercourse. Their orientation during the sexual act is primarily the attainment of an orgasm. Women on the other hand need about twenty to thirty minutes of foreplay to get sexually excited. They are more interested in affection, in being hugged with tenderness, in tactile caresses of the body, in being loved in a nonsexual way. This is a very important part of triggering the woman's desire to be possessed. Foreplay allows her to feel loved and helps her relax and enjoy the sexual act.

It is very difficult for a woman to have an orgasm if she does not participate in sexual foreplay. Men may misinterpret the fact that women do no get excited as quickly as they do. The fact that a woman needs more time devoted to foreplay does not mean that she is not interested in making love. She just needs more time to get ready. This is why foreplay is essential in order for the woman to have an orgasm.

A woman needs to satisfy her emotional needs before she can fully participate in lovemaking. Men must be aware of this need, especially if the woman has had an intense working day and has been busy with other chores. She needs to relax and feel loved, not to be used as a sexual object.

When sexual dissatisfaction becomes chronic, a woman will develop a negative attitude towards the sexual act, even if the interpersonal relationship is adequate. If the relationship deteriorates, it may be due not so much to sexual dissatisfaction as to the feeling that the woman's emotional needs are not met by the man's inadequate attitude during foreplay.

The man may occasionally doubt that his partner has reached orgasm since the woman sometimes pretends that she has so as not to disappoint him. If the man is experienced enough and can detect when the woman simulates an orgasm, she may develop a sense of guilt and depression.

It cannot be emphasized enough that the man must recognize that a woman is very different from him in this respect as well as in others. She can experience more pleasure without always having an orgasm, if the man takes the necessary time to express his affection during foreplay.

Drinking alcohol prior to the sexual act may cause the inability to reach a climax. In other circumstances, alcohol and drugs in particular may make it difficult to maintain an erection.

The percentage of women who reach a climax is lower than that of men. It is important to be acquainted with the factors that conspire against the attainment of a climax by women so that the deterioration of the couple's relationship can be avoided.

We have mentioned that women have two areas whose stimulation can produce a climax. One is the tactile or oral stimulation of the clitoris; the other is the anterior wall of the external third of the vagina when stimulated by the penis.

During intercourse the clitoris is practically not stimulated by the penis. Some people believe that during vaginal penetration some of the structures that cover the clitoris are elongated, which would cause it to be stimulated, and that this stimulus would be reinforced by the contraction of the ischio cavernous muscles, which are located in the bulb of the clitoris that is attached to the ischium of the pubic bone.

Women are categorical in describing that vaginal pleasure starts at the upper anterior third of the vagina, a sensation that is intensified by intercourse in certain positions and by the contraction of the bulbocavernous muscles that increase the friction of the penis when entering the vagina. They can also distinguish very clearly the pleasure derived from stimulation of the clitoris from that originating in the vagina.

Despite the wide dissemination of sexual material that has flooded the press, the movies, music, and other communication media since 1960, the educational value of this information for a better understanding of women's sexuality is questionable.

Ignorance, myths and taboos, and the effect of sexual trauma caused by rape and sexual abuse during childhood and puberty, play a negative role in the development of sexuality and the actualization of a normal sexual experience in adult women.

Lack of acquaintance with their own anatomy and physiology is such that many women have never masturbated and would not know how to do it. Those who have experienced orgasm by any means, including masturbation, are more likely to reach orgasm with their partners when married.

Few women have an orgasm on their first sexual relation. Furthermore many women have never had an orgasm during ten or more years of matrimony. Very few women learn to voluntarily contact the bulbocavernous muscles to increase the friction by the penis on the vagina. These are powerful muscles. The woman who does not want or fears vaginal penetration may make entrance by the penis practically impossible. This is observed in those cases of vaginism where the bulbocavernous muscles remain in a state of spasm, voluntary or unconscious.

Hormones play an important role in the awakening of sexual desire and the ability to reach a climax. In animals there is a close relation between hormonal levels, sexual desire, and sexual response. In humans this relation is not as close. In women hormonal level affects sexual response only when hormonal levels are abnormal.

The effect of the menstrual cycle on sexual behavior is very imprecise. Some studies reveal that sexual desire and sexual response increase slightly during the days close to ovulation (day 15) and during the 22nd to the 26th day of the menstrual period. In women suffering from a painful pre-menstrual syndrome this increase does not occur. The feeling of discomfort takes precedence over any other hormonal effect of the cycle.

Another hormonal aspect to consider is the effect of oral contraceptives on the sexual response of women. Some women note that the sensitivity of their breasts increases while under the effect of contraceptives while their sexual desire and pleasure diminish. For others, this effect may be minimal or nonexistent. This may depend on the type of oral contraceptive that is used.

Intrauterine contraceptives cause uncomfortable uterine contractions and abdominal pain during orgasm in 10 to 20 percent of women, but in the majority of the cases these devices do not interfere with arousal and orgasm.

Diaphragms and spermatocides produce an uncomfortable sensation and genital irritation during intercourse for some women. Others find that antispermatic creams produce an excess of lubrication that diminishes sexual pleasure. Psychologically the fact that a diaphragm must be inserted prior to intercourse inhibits the spontaneity of the sexual act.

The use of condoms in general reduces sensitivity and inhibits spontaneity both for men and women. Condoms made of natural materials transmit heat and sensation better than latex condoms.

Other methods of contraception, such as following the ovulatory rhythm or practicing coitus interruptus, are quite marginal as far as their effectiveness in preventing pregnancy. Besides, these methods greatly inhibit the spontaneity of the sexual act.

Sterilization of the man or the woman is an ideal method of contraception for couples that do not want to have more than two or three children. Under these conditions, sexual desire and orgasm are not affected and the sexual act is totally spontaneous.

The effect of age on the capacity to respond sexually depends on psychological and physical factors. If a woman thinks she will become less sexual as she grows old it is likely that she will feel less sexual and her sexual response will diminish, but this will be mainly for psychological reasons.

Decrease in the sexual response of women is in great part due to a cultural myth, as shown by the research of Alfred Kinsley during the 50's. He found that women's sexuality reaches its peak in their late thirties, after which it declines slightly. There are some physical changes at this age that may affect sexuality, but they are not significant enough to reduce sexual pleasure if the woman is aware of these changes.

Age-related changes in women's sexuality are associated with the reduction of female hormones, mainly estrogen, in the ovaries. This reduction starts around age 45 and continues throughout menopause until approximately age 55 on the average. After this period, hormonal level stays relatively stable.

With the reduction of estrogen come various changes that may affect sexual responses: the vaginal mucous membrane becomes thinner, less moist, and more likely to become irritated during intercourse; vaginal lubrication, which at an earlier age would start within thirty seconds of the initiation of sexual activity, may now take from three to five minutes and be insufficient to allow an older woman to enjoy the sexual act; the clitoris may become less sensitive and change in size.

Furthermore, the skin becomes less sensitive to touch, and caresses may not be as pleasant as they used to be at an earlier age. Orgasmic contractions, which may include spasmodic contractions of the uterus, may become more painful than pleasant.

The muscle tone of the urinary tract may also be influenced by estrogen. Some women may lose a small amount of urine during orgasm. These changes may be small for the majority of women and their effects may not be as devastating as one would imagine. Doses of estrogen combined with progesterone are common practice for women with sexual problems deriving from menopause and aging.

When this hormonal combination is periodically discontinued, the woman may have a menstrual period, but the risk of developing uterine cervical cancer or breast cancer is minimal, since progesterone significantly reduces this possibility. The combined use of estrogen and progesterone also reduces the risk of heart illness and osteoporosis, which are common at this age.

Hysterectomy, which sometimes involves removal of the ovaries and is performed for medical reasons, creates a "surgical menopause", with the same potential effects on sexuality as natural menopause. The administration of combined hormones, estrogen and progesterone, controls this problem satisfactorily.

There is a great number of medical substances that have a negative influence on sexual response. Drugs intended to control anxiety, depression and insomnia lower sexual desire, inhibit sexual arousal, and interfere with orgasm.

Additionally, various drugs intended to treat cardiac problems, arterial hypertension, and digestive ulcers may have similar negative effects for some women.

The substance that most commonly interferes with sexual response and desire is alcohol, contrary to the common belief that alcohol reduces inhibition and heightens sexual response. The psychological effect of drinking a glass of wine may appear to be one of relaxation at the beginning, but further drinking interferes with sexual arousal and orgasm for women.

It is normal to experience a temporal reduction of interest in sex due to stress at work, loss of a loved one, loss of a job, or any other circumstance that makes one of the partners not to feel well. What matters in these cases is that the lack of interest in sex has nothing to do with the interpersonal relation of the couple.

In other cases the choice of the moment to make love may be inappropriate for one of the partners. For instance, the husband may want to make love in the morning when the wife needs to get up to go to work. Her lack of interest may be misinterpreted as lack of consideration and respect for her partner. The repetition of this pattern may indicate that some emotional need is not being met.

When the couple is in the bedroom engaged in passionate foreplay, one must be careful not to do something inappropriate that may interrupt or inhibit the moment's passion and romance. Inappropriate behavior or conversation, such as saying something that may be hurtful, is clearly out of the context of the romantic situation. It is advisable that any discussion or argument take place outside the bedroom. Otherwise the love nest becomes a battlefield that in time can only destroy the couple's harmony.

It is important for the man to be delicate in initiating and performing the sexual act, especially the first time that his partner has sex. For fear of penetration by the penis the woman may involuntarily contract her muscles and thus make vaginal penetration difficult and painful. The man must try to prolong his caresses, and delay penetration until the woman gains confidence and relaxes. If this is not possible, the man should wait and either try again or let the woman adopt a position where she can control the movement and penetration of the penis. Rudeness and aggressiveness on the part of the man is not necessary and counterproductive. At any rate, friction of the glans when entering a narrow vagina is very pleasurable for the man and allows for a satisfactory ejaculation and orgasm.

The obsessive tendency to focus only on getting an orgasm interferes with the spontaneity of the sexual act. This is most often the case when the man suffers from premature ejaculation, which is also a frequent cause of the woman not having an orgasm during intercourse. On the one hand, the man is worried about not reaching the crucial moment when ejaculation can no longer be controlled. On the other, the woman focuses her attention on limiting the expression of her desire, slowing down the rhythm of her movement so as to avoid reaching the point of no return when ejaculation is inevitable. In these cases the most appropriate procedure is to concentrate on caressing each other keeping the rhythm of penetration as slow as possible and stopping as soon as the man feels the onset of pleasure. It is preferable to let the woman control penetration and movement in these situations.

Because of fear of premature ejaculation or not being able to maintain an erection to satisfy his partner, the man is incapable of controlling a mechanism that is completely involuntary. When the situation repeats itself over and over again it gives rise to a conditioned reflex which can only be changed by altering the conditions and time of stimulation or varying the aim of the sexual act by placing more emphasis on the expression of love and affection than on physical pleasure.

Sexual desire and response decrease or disappear when physical attraction diminishes due to bodily changes, insufficient genital cleanliness, or offensive odors. Appropriate mutual hygiene is very important. Showering together and lathering each other's bodies with a soft massage of the genitals is a good stimulant.

If sexual attraction is the major component of an interpersonal relation, the decrease or absence of sexual desire is reason enough for the relationship to come to an end.

An increase of prolactin in the blood serum, which occurs right after pregnancy and has the function of stimulating the breasts for the purpose of milk secretion, inhibits sexual desire. Furthermore, high levels of prolactin in women produces amenorrhea, loss of vaginal lubrication and consequently pain during intercourse. For men, an increase in prolactin due to a tumor in the pituitary gland inhibits sexual desire.

Malfunction of the thyroid also affects sexual desire and erection. Various drugs used to control gastric ulcers, hypertension, or to treat anxiety and depression inhibit sexual desire and interfere with the reaching of an orgasm. Some of these effects are secondary results of the increase of prolactin caused by the medications themselves. In men, sexual interest and desire is also negatively affected by lack of production of testosterone.

Women may learn how to reach an orgasm, but negative cultural and religious influences may still inhibit sexual desire. They may feel embarrassed or guilty about initiating sexual activity with their partners or about stimulating themselves. Other women may have unpleasant reactions during intercourse due to the activation of strong emotions caused by traumatic sexual experiences in their childhood, adolescence or adulthood, such as abuse or rape.

Some women who are capable of having orgasms are afraid to be carried away by sexual desire and lose control. The fear to become insatiable, immoral, and loose, may automatically suppress or inhibit their sexual desire. They should understand that having sexual desires and reaching an orgasm does not make them different persons. One does not become a different person unless one wishes to do so.

Mental depression, slight or severe, is also recognized as an inhibiting factor of sexual desire. Symptoms of depression include feelings of regret, lack of self-esteem, low levels of energy, insomnia, and lack of appetite.

The couple's life style is important. It is unreasonable to expect having sexual desires if one is chronically tired and stressed. If the couple is not happy, the sexual desire is also at risk. It is common for a woman to experience lack of sexual desire when she feels that her partner is domineering and despotic, that there is no give and take, and decisions are not made by mutual agreement.

Some women experience inhibition of sexual desire due to fear of being vulnerable to their partners. Making love is a sign of deep affection for your partner and is associated with the perceived need to satisfy him emotionally. This should be a pleasant emotion, but it may turn into fear if the woman cannot trust her partner to be there for her when she needs him. These feelings may be observed in women from families where the mother was abused by the father or in women who have had bad experiences in previous relationships. They may try to have sexual desires but they can't.

A sexual relation is an expression of love and affection as well as a form of play. Men and women driven by an intense need to work who have a strict sense of responsibility oriented towards success in the form of making more money than others, having the smartest children and the most elegant houses may find it difficult to acknowledge their more frivolous and playful selves and get in touch with their sexual desires. They may then relegate sex to the lowest priority as the least important and desirable activity. In time, the enjoyment of a sexual relation diminishes and the motivation to engage in sex disappears.

Fantasy is part of sexual expression. It may increase the sexual response and pleasure of a couple. It is important that both partners feel comfortable with the idea of using fantasy to augment sexual response. Fantasy allows us to imagine making love in a variety of circumstances or situations, many of which will never take place in the real world. Fantasy provides heightened interest, allows us to satisfy our curiosity, at the same time protecting us from doing something that we would rather not do.

Both partners must understand the significance of using fantasy while making love. They must also think about how the use of fantasy may affect their relationship. A woman may feel that it is wrong or false to imagine making love with somebody other than her partner, since he may think that he is incapable of satisfying her sexually. Some women, however, can only be aroused by imagining sex with somebody other than their partner.

Some studies show that more than 50 percent of married women have sexual fantasies, at least occasionally, while having sex with their partners. Some women may have sexual dreams even when they are not doing anything sexual. They are usually people with imagination and creativity. Most of the women who have sexual fantasies enjoy them and have satisfying sexual relations with their partners.

Of course the content of fantasies varies considerably from one person to another. Many women include their partners in their fantasies but change the location (on the beach, at a party, in the shower, or in a cabin in the woods, to cite some examples). They may also change the number of people involved (orgies, swapping of partners) or imagine other types of activity (whipping, aggression, submission). Others imagine these situations without their partners.

What matters is that fantasies have a positive effect on the sexual relation of the couple. Fantasies stimulate sensations, they make women feel more sexual, and this heightened sexual desire makes them want to share something that their partners may also enjoy.

Fantasies may help a woman focus on sexual pleasure instead of worrying about what has happened during the day or what will happen the next day. They may help trigger a woman's sexual desire and arousal without her partner having to do it all.

It must be kept in mind that as we grow up and discover the significance of sexuality what we are taught about sex is that it is something forbidden. It shouldn't surprise us then that many people want to retain that forbidden element and include part of the fantasy in their lovemaking.

If fantasies are perceived to have a negative effect on the relationship it is advisable to talk to the couple. It may be that they are both interested in using fantasies during the process of stimulation, not just during intercourse.

It may be possible to decide not to share one's fantasy entirely with one's partner, since keeping it secret makes it very special. What is important, though, is to communicate to one's partner this decision and assure him or her that the fantasy increases sexuality and has a positive influence on the evolution of the couple as such.

When sharing a fantasy with one's partner one must be careful not to include in it some other person that he or she might know. Although many people do not mind that their partner may fantasize about having sex with a movie star or the centerfold of some magazine, they might become jealous if their partner has sexual fantasies involving somebody they both know. If one has that type of fantasy it might be advisable not to share it with one's partner or clarify that it is just a fantasy, not a real desire to have sex with that person. It is normal to be sexually attracted to somebody other than one's partner, but that does not mean that one will act on that attraction.

Let us remember that not having sexual fantasies before or during intercourse is also normal. What matters is that each participant keep focused on his or her own physical pleasure and that of his or her partner, since sharing is pleasurable for both.

This general review of the causes and factors that interfere with sexual arousal and the attainment of orgasm shows that this is more common in women than in men, and this explains the high percentage of women who cannot have an orgasm.

If we factor out the physiological, hormonal, psychological, and medical causes, we find that the predominant factors responsible for the sexual dissatisfaction of couples are lack of education, ignorance of the sexual function, and the fragility of some interpersonal relations.

One should analyze the real factors that have led to the establishment of an interpersonal relation. In many cases the relationship is based only on physical and sexual attraction, while other factors, like communication, the ability to share common interests, the existence of an affective bond, the vision of clear goals, are very superficial or fragile.

Knowledge of human sexuality is important, since it allows the members of a couple to have a better understanding of their function as individuals and as partners. In practice this kind of education is very precarious, with incomplete and distorted information.

Having these facts into account, one can conclude that for many couples with a satisfactory interpersonal relation, an important cause of sexual dissatisfaction of the woman is premature ejaculation by her partner. The inappropriate conduct of the man, who in many cases is culturally conditioned to take the initiative leading to making love, is one of the major factors preventing his partner from reaching orgasm. Foreplay is generally limited and predictable, not allowing the woman to prepare herself physically and psychologically.

On the other hand, if the interpersonal relation is unsatisfactory and one's emotional needs are not met, the sexual act will also be unsatisfactory for one of the members of the couple, most likely the woman. This is why we emphasize the importance of a lasting interpersonal relation based on good communication, participation and mutual appreciation.

Kegel's Vaginal Exercises

In 1952 Dr. Arnold Kegel described some special exercises for the muscles of the female urogenital zone. These muscles include the surface perineal transverse, the bulbocavernous, the ischiocavernous, the deep perineal transverse, and the urethral sphincter. These exercises were originally designed to treat urinary incontinence in women. It has been well established that a good muscular tone of these muscles may not only increase most women's ability to reach orgasm but also to intensify it. Some women, however, are unable to reach orgasm in spite of the strength of these muscles, which may be due to other causes.

The vaginal exercises described by Dr. Arnold Kegel are intended to improve the muscular tone of the muscles just mentioned, in particular the bulbocavernous and the ischiocavernous muscles. Maintaining a good contraction and muscle tone facilitates the friction of the penis with the vaginal wall. This stimulates the nerve endings of the vaginal mucous membrane, especially the external upper third that includes the area next to the entrance to the vagina that is surrounded by the erectile tissue of the vestibular bulb and by the muscular fibers of the bulbocavernous muscle. Besides improving muscle tone, these exercises facilitate the blood flow to the erectile tissue of the bulbocavernous muscle increasing the sexual sensation and the ability to get an orgasm. Muscle contraction involving additional pelvic muscles increases the blood flow in the pelvic region, facilitating sexual arousal and intensifying orgasm. Once the woman starts feeling a pleasant sensation in her genitals, she can concentrate on it without worrying only about whether she will or will not get an orgasm. It is useful to experience all these pleasant sensations and share them with one's partner. Adequate stimulation of the penis also increases the man's pleasure.

The effects of these exercises are more noticeable in women who have had children and women over 40, particularly if they have lived a sedentary life without exercise.

In order to recognize and feel the muscle contraction during these exercises it is necessary to concentrate one's attention on the final stage of emptying one's bladder when urinating. When a woman stops urinating, her bladder's sphincter contracts, and she is aware of this function. Contraction of the other pelvic muscles does not initially produce the same sensation because they are too weak.

DIRECTIONS FOR VAGINAL EXERCISES

1. Lie in bed on your back, or sit on a chair.

2. Breathe deeply, hold your breath for 3 seconds and contract your muscles the way you do when you stop urinating. Exhale and relax your muscles. At first, the abdominal muscles may participate. To obtain the desired sensation more easily, contract also your hip muscles (gluteal region) while raising your pelvis.

3. Repeat these exercises 30 times per session.

4. You can also do the exercises every time you urinate.

5. Concentrate on the sensation you feel during the exercises.

6. Choose the place where you can best relax and concentrate on what you are doing.

7. You can also do the exercises during intercourse while your partner's penis is in your vagina.

8. These exercises must be done twice a day during your whole sexually active life.

Oral Sex

It would have been impossible to discuss this topic thirty years ago. Despite the expanded sexual information we have today, the subject is full of taboos, ignorance and superstition so that its practice has caused much suffering especially for women.

Historically, oral sex is as old as humanity itself. In the Egyptian papyri dating back to 1700 BC there are references to it. Similarly in the literature, paintings, and sculptures of ancient Greece, Rome, India, and Japan. There are historical accounts to the effect that native American women from Cuba practiced it with Spanish conquistadors, who were crazy about this type of erotic stimulation. From a biological point of view, this practice is part of our philogenetic heredity, it being a common practice among different mammal species. Comparative studies of human sexual behavior have shown that oral sex is part of most human societies and that it is only in the Western world, dominated by the Judeo-Christian tradition, that the practice of this technique of sexual satisfaction has not been easily adopted. Western religions prohibit it and in some countries like England and the United States it is considered illegal. There have been cases where a man was condemned to life in prison for having practiced oral sex with his own wife. In other cases, women who have consented to practice oral sex with their husbands and have subsequently divorced have accused their husbands of sexual perversion, denying that they had ever consented to such practice. In the United States, according to the studies of Dr. Alfred Kinsey, 95% of men and 75% of women practice oral sex. The existence of archaic legislation, taboos, religious pressure, and ignorance, however, produce anxiety, fear, and apprehension in married couples that doubt whether oral stimulation or sex is good or bad. This creates an emotional conflict that may affect the relationship and the sexual function of the couple. In order to prevent conflict caused by the practice of oral sex, it is important for the couple to act without inhibitions, restrictions, or sense of guilt, and treat it as an expression of mutual love.

Oral sex is self-defining: it is the oral stimulation of the male or female sexual organs. Stimulation of the female genitals, specifically the labia majora and minora of the vulva and the clitoris, by the man's lips and tongue is called cunnilingus. Stimulation of the penis by the woman's mouth is called fellatio.

According to Dr. Alfred Kinsey's studies, at least 50% of married men and women have practiced oral sex. The percentage is higher among young and educated couples. Among lower and uneducated classes, its practice is less common, due to the prevailing taboos against it. In casual sexual encounters, oral sex is very common.

In cunnilingus the man must place himself between the open legs of the woman, facing her and with his head against the vulva and clitoris. The best procedure for the man is to apply his lips and tongue to the woman's external genitals while she lies on her back, her hips at the edge of the bed and raised by pillows, and her legs separated and bent. This allows a better contact of her thighs with the man's face, a better separation of the labia majora, and better exposure of the clitoris. Tongue stimulation must be slow and soft at the beginning, to allow erection of the clitoris. Once the woman starts to react, the rhythm of stimulation may be increased. The man must always remember that that sexual zone of the woman is very sensitive and delicate. Any roughness may totally inhibit the woman's sexual excitement.

In fellatio, the woman places herself between the man's open legs, facing him with her head right above his abdomen, to facilitate penetration of the penis. There are several variants of this position. Under one of them, the man lies on his back with his hips at the edge of the bed and the woman kneels in front of him. This is a very comfortable position for the woman . Another variant has the man sitting on a chair and the woman kneeling in front of him. This position facilitates stimulation by the tongue of the lower part of the glans and the frenulum, which is the most sensitive area to tactile stimulation. To increase the sensibility of the penis during fellatio, the woman may use one of her hands to retract the prepuce and squeeze the penis between the thumb and the index as a kind of ring around the body of the penis. Retraction of the prepuce and pressure applied to the penis at the moment of orgasm significantly increases the man's sexual pleasure.

The penis need not totally penetrate the woman's mouth. All that is needed for adequate stimulation is for the woman to keep the glans and the area right behind it in her mouth. This way, her lips stimulate the glans crown, and her tongue stimulates the lower part of the penis, especially the frenulum and its surrounding area. By keeping the prepuce retracted with her thumb and index, she exposes the most sensitive area of the penis to oral contact during the movements of penetration and withdrawal.

It is advisable for both the man and the woman to keep their genitals clean, to prevent a reaction of displeasure caused by an offensive odor. If this is routinely attended to, there is no reason for the smell or taste of secretions to be unpleasant.

Most couples practice oral sex as part of foreplay prior to intercourse. Other couples do it as a form of satisfaction or to prevent pregnancy. A woman may have several orgasms during oral stimulation of the clitoris. Men, on the other hand, are not multi orgasmic. Once orgasm is achieved, the penis returns to its flaccid state for a variable period of time, after which stimulation may produce another erection.

Most men like to ejaculate inside a woman's mouth, but some women find it unpleasant, at least the first few times. Other women, however, find it strongly exciting and may reach an orgasm at that instant. In order to prevent reactions of displeasure, couples should discuss openly whether they like or not this type of sexual stimulation. If the woman has had a painful experience with oral sex, she will understandably feel uncomfortable about practicing it. The most common reason of displeasure or rejection of oral sex on the part of the woman is the idea that it is somehow dirty and that practicing it is humiliating and immoral.

The seminal liquid, as explained in a previous chapter, consists of sperm secreted by the testicles, the prostate, the urethral glands, and the seminal vesicles. This mix takes place during intercourse and is completed at the moment of ejaculation. It resembles saliva in its appearance and consistency. It is somewhat acid to the taste and it has a penetrating smell. Knowing these facts may help eliminate some erroneous ideas about oral sex.

As part of foreplay, oral stimulation is very important, not only for the emotional intensity involved but also because it allows the woman to awaken the sexual sensations that will help her get an orgasm. Its practice provides each member of the couple the opportunity to express his or her affection, consideration, delicacy, and tenderness. Besides, the desire to share all kinds of pleasant sensations in an intimate physical and emotional union leads to the realization and integration of a sense of mutual love.

As for the ability to practice oral sex, it does not require a special technique. What matters is the desire to do it and the pleasure it affords both members of the couple. Some women feel awkward and lacking initiative, but this can be corrected with experience and by asking their partners what they like and what excites them the most. Women may also complain about men's roughness during oral sex.

The most common causes that inhibit or interfere with the spontaneity of oral sex are the idea that the practice is dirty, sinful, perverted, or the fact that it evokes an unpleasant memory. It is possible that an uninhibited woman may show more initiative and creativity during fellatio than the man during cunnilingus.

In cases of sexual impotence or premature ejaculation by the man, oral sex with a slow rhythm may be very satisfying for a man with erection problems, particularly when the problem is psychological. The woman may temporarily interrupt the stimulation and thus delay ejaculation. This way the man may gradually gain confidence and be able to achieve orgasm during intercourse. In this kind of situation it is important for the woman to play an active role, placing herself on top of the man, who lies on his back while the woman controls vaginal penetration.

The woman's participation in the treatment of premature ejaculation is very important. Oral stimulation of the penis must be slow while keeping the prepuce retracted with her thumb and index and applying pressure to the body of the penis, interrupting oral stimulation as soon

as the man signals that he is getting close to orgasm. After a one-
or two-minute pause, she starts a new cycle. After five to ten cycles,
there may be vaginal penetration with the woman playing an active
role as described above. This technique must be used every time there
is sexual intercourse.

Under certain circumstances there may be transmission of venereal
diseases. The existence of a lesion in the oral cavity may allow the
presence of germs in the epithelium of the oral membrane. There
is no difference between cunnilingus and fellatio with respect to
the danger of venereal infection. Herpes may be transmitted during
cunnilingus, as well vaginal or urethral infection due to severe cases
of staphylococci and streptococci. Gonorrhea is less likely to be
transmitted during oral sex than syphilis.

As for the transmission of the virus responsible for AIDS there
is insufficient information. It has been shown that in monkeys the
infection may occur through the oral mucous membrane without
there being any lesions.

Although there is no indication that AIDS may be transmitted in
humans through mouth-to-mouth contact by kissing, sharing utensils,
etc., it is possible that infection may occur. One study shows that oral
infection may occur doses 6,000 times smaller than the dose needed
to cause rectal infection during anal sex. Studies provide strong
evidence that oral ejaculation by an infected man may cause AIDS
even if the virus is swallowed. Similarly, fellatio with a condom is
not one hundred percent safe if the man has the AIDS virus.

Anal Sex

Sexual satisfaction through penetration of the penis in your partner's anus, so-called 'coitus against nature', is common practice among homosexuals, but it also occurs in heterosexual relations, although it is not as common. We must admit that it is satisfying for men. There are men who emphatically claim that the only way they can get an erection is when they practice anal intercourse. Without getting into a complex explanation of the psychological dynamics of anal intercourse, it is clear that some sociocultural factors play a determining role. We are all familiar with the hostile, aggressive, and humiliating verbal insults with a sexual content concerning the anal area. You could say that for a man practicing it is an expression of dominance, whereas for a woman it expresses submission.

Most women are afraid to engage in it, but for some it is wholly satisfying and they even prefer it to vaginal penetration. The main concern is the size of the penis. Those women that prefer anal sex practice it without fear as long as the diameter of the penis is small. Although what we have said so far relates only to the psychological aspect of sexual desire, there are some other factors that must be taken into account.

From the anatomical and physiological point of view, the nerve composition of the anal region is identical to that of the vagina, since in both cases the somatic and neurovegetative nerves originate in the same segments of the spine. Because of this, the possibility that a woman may feel a pleasant sensation and even have an orgasm during anal intercourse has an anatomical and physiological basis.

It is important to know that the epithelium of the rectal mucous membrane is entirely different from and lacks the firmness of the vaginal membrane. Consequently it is more easily hurt during penetration by the penis, causing painful and bleeding anal fissures that may be infected. On the other hand, the microbial flora of the rectum is rich and infectious. It is advisable for those who practice this mode of sexual satisfaction to use latex condoms and plenty of lubrication with a non-water soluble lubricant like vaseline. Penetration must be slow and it must be stopped if there is pain. There should never be vaginal penetration right after anal insertion. To do this is an invitation to vaginal infection by the rectal bacterial flora, which may have serious consequences. People suffering from hemorrhoids should not practice anal intercourse.

Some men practice anal penetration at the moment of ejaculation as a way to prevent pregnancy. The fact that penetration is brief does not prevent the complications mentioned above or the possibility of HIV infection.

Premature Ejaculation

This sexual dysfunction constitutes one of the most common causes of female sexual dissatisfaction, especially in couples who plan to live together for a long time, married or otherwise.

The expression 'premature ejaculation' indicates that ejaculation occurs a short time after the penis is stimulated. According to C. Armes, 8% of men suffer from erectile dysfunction, and 30% of those men suffer from premature ejaculation. A study of 100 normal couples varying in age from 30 to 40, an age of intense sexual activity when 90% of the couples consider themselves happy, showed that 36 men suffered from premature ejaculation. From these studies we can conclude that premature ejaculation is one of the most common sexual dysfunctions, especially among men under 50.

It is hard to define premature ejaculation, as there is no agreement concerning the time that must elapse between stimulation of the penis and ejaculation.

Masters and Johnson leave out of consideration the time factor and define premature ejaculation in terms of a woman's satisfaction during intercourse. If the woman fails to be satisfied 50% of the time, they determine that the man suffers from premature ejaculation. If we take into account that a woman needs 20 to 30 minutes of foreplay and at least 15 minutes of intercourse, any ejaculation that occurs before this time must be considered premature. The definition itself implies ejaculation in a short period of time probably under five minutes. We must remember that men reach a climax much sooner than women.

There are men who ejaculate during foreplay, before vaginal penetration or right after having their penis penetrate the vagina. The definition itself is not important if the man and his partner know what is happening. What matters is that this form of sexual dysfunction is one of the major causes of female dissatisfaction in marriage. A woman without much information may tolerate it for some time, but she may find out from other women that this is not normal. The man may also lack the relevant information as to how to stimulate his partner during foreplay, and he may blame her for "lack of concentration" to achieve orgasm. Most women in this situation lack the necessary strength to suggest to their husbands that they should seek professional help. Some women may not want to hurt their partner, so they fail to raise the topic with him.

Premature ejaculation may be due to a variety of causes. For better understanding we have divided them as follows:

1. Organic causes. These included pathologies affecting the sacral nervous system, heightened sensitivity of the penis, the prostate or the urethra. In general it is unlikely for premature ejaculation to be the only symptom of lesions in these organs. It is useful to have a good medical history and examination of the genitals and the rectum plus a neurological exam.

2. Behavioral causes. Premature ejaculation usually starts at an early stage of sexual awakening, including masturbation. Given the information they receive, most young men consider masturbation as something abnormal and therefore forbidden. For fear of being caught in the act, young men masturbate in bed or other places that offer protection from others. For this reason they masturbate as fast as possible in order to get an orgasm. The repetition of this behavior produces a conditioned reflex that shortens the time between stimulus and ejaculation. We must remember that when a man masturbates, ejaculation occurs in less than five minutes.

Similarly, sexual contact with prostitutes requires the sexual act to be as short as possible, since they are not interested in their own climax during the sexual act. Intercourse in an uncomfortable position, like the back seat of a car or a place where there is a risk of being caught, leads to reducing the interval between stimulus and ejaculation to the shortest possible time. Finally, the fear of impotence may lead to premature ejaculation when having sex for the first time.

3. Psychological causes. The husband sometimes starts worrying about his condition due to his wife's complaints, but the problem subsists due to his fear of not being able to control ejaculation. The

main reason for this is poor communication between husband and wife. He must acknowledge his problem and she must understand that what happens is beyond his voluntary control and in no way signals lack of consideration on his part.

In some rare cases the problem arises when the man fears he might be impotent or when he is forced into a sexual relation that he is not interested in. Other common factors are insecurity and fear to fail or to be rejected for not being physically attractive.

Some authors believe that the conflicts at home that young people witness may result in this type of dysfunction when they become adults. Additionally, lack of independence and security plus possible negative consequences of sexual awakening during childhood may affect a man's sexuality in the future. I do not believe that sexual traumatic experiences may be responsible for premature ejaculation, although they may to some extent constitute the psychological mechanism for impotence.

TREATMENT

The treatment of premature ejaculation must be based on the mechanism responsible for it. Taking into account that its causes are primarily behavioral and psychological, we could outline its mechanism as follows:

Physiologically speaking, we must remember that penile erection is a function of the autonomous parasympathetic nervous system. Ejaculation and return to a flaccid state are under the control of the autonomous sympathetic nervous system. The latter is activated as a result of the discharge of norepinephrine leading to constriction of the arteries and muscles of the corpora cavernosa of the penis after ejaculation.

Based on the neurophysiological model of the mechanism of stress, the anxiety associated with masturbation produces ejaculation within a short period of time. There seems to be a low threshold of excitation or a condition of hyperactivity of the secondary autonomous nervous system under stress.

If in the future the subject faces the sexual act with anxiety, he will experience the same conditions. The final result will be premature ejaculation.

Later on, his fear to fail, his insecurity, and the sense of not being able to control ejaculation will trigger the discharge of norepinephrine, with the result described above. Some men deny the existence of anxiety, and yet continue to have the same problem.

Essentially, a conditioned reflex is created by the repetition of its components: external stimulation, anxiety, discharge of norepinephrine, ejaculation.

The goal of treatment of premature ejaculation is to achieve conscious control of the external stimuli of erection, and to prevent any attempt to exercise voluntary control over ejaculation.

The treatment should begin during foreplay, the stage where genitals are caressed, and specifically the penis is manually or orally stimulated. As soon as the man feels a sensation of pleasure, foreplay is stopped until the sensation disappears. After repeating this cycle five to ten times, the man can ejaculate. Once he achieves a certain measure of control, he can attempt intercourse in certain positions: the man lies on his back and the woman sits on top of him and controls penetration with back and forth movements of her hips. Again, as soon as he experiences a sensation of pleasure, she stops her movement until the sensation disappears. The process is repeated five to ten times, and then he is allowed to ejaculate. It is advisable to repeat this sexual act at least three times a week without necessarily reaching a climax every time.

A variant of this position may be used where the man uses an anesthetic cream around the glans and frenulum, and a condom to prevent the cream from affecting the vagina. The position and control of penetration and movement by the woman remains the same as above.

This position is very satisfying for the woman, since it produces friction of the penis on the upper area of the external third of the vagina, which is her most sensitive area. It is best for this practice to occur with full cooperation from both partners.

For single men who have no constant sexual partner and engage in casual encounters, the procedure for breaking the conditioned reflex must be different. Masturbation provides one opportunity to achieve non-voluntary control of ejaculation. The manual stimulation of the penis must proceed slowly and stop as soon as a sensation of pleasure is felt. This cycle must be repeated five to ten times, after which the man may ejaculate, if he so desires.

The variant using an anesthetic cream and a condom is also recommended. Masturbation with or without the use of an anesthetic must be repeated daily without necessarily reaching orgasm.

In the future, when the single man has a steady sexual partner, he must explain his situation to her and establish good communication to obtain her cooperation and have a sexual experience in an environment of relaxation and harmony. It is important to establish that every time he has a sexual relation he must proceed the same way until he achieves involuntary control over the time between stimulus and ejaculation.

The practice of these methods requires frequent repetition for an optimal result. This is based on the physiological fact that stimuli lose their effectiveness when their frequency increases. For this reason, it is advisable that whenever possible the practice occur on a daily basis. For couples this could be limited to foreplay, mainly involving manual or oral stimulation of the penis as indicated above. If the couple wants to have intercourse after foreplay, this must be done in the same way described before.

Once the man has achieved involuntary control of ejaculation, he can try other positions for intercourse, provided they give the woman satisfactory stimulation. The following position is recommended: The woman lies on her back and the man on his left side. The woman's right leg is flexed and rests on the man's right leg. The man crosses his right leg over the woman's extended left leg (like scissors). Once vaginal penetration is accomplished, the man stimulates the woman's clitoris with the middle finger of his right hand. In this position, the man's exertion is minimal, and the woman has vaginal stimulation by the penis plus manual stimulation of the clitoris. The man carries on the back and forth movement of penetration at the same time that he stimulates his partner's clitoris. As soon as he feels the onset of a sensation of pleasure, he stops penetration until the sensation disappears, but continues stimulation of the clitoris. This cycle is repeated five to ten times. When the woman reacts to stimulation of the clitoris and the vagina and is about to reach a climax, the man resumes penetration by the penis and can ejaculate during the woman's climax or afterward. With some experience the man will be able to detect the contraction of the woman's vaginal muscles during climax. It is not good for the man to reach a climax before the woman since the penis will return to its flaccid state, which in all probability with interfere with the woman's progress towards orgasm.

The Masters and Johnson technique known as the "squeeze technique" consists of manual stimulation of the penis by the woman. As soon as the man starts feeling pleasure, the woman stops the procedure, after which she applies pressure to the frenulum with the tip of her thumb and to the back of the glans with her index, in a back and forth direction, never laterally, for about four seconds. It is important that the woman use her fingertips, not her nails, so as not to harm the penis's skin. The rationale is the same as explained before, that is, to try to break the conditioned reflex in order to prolong the time between stimulus and ejaculation.

The woman repeats the procedure five times before allowing penetration. Once the man's penis is inside the vagina, it is recommended that both partners stay still for fifteen to thirty seconds, before starting slow movement of the penis. It is advisable to practice this technique daily if possible, without necessarily reaching orgasm even if there has been vaginal penetration.

Another alternative is the use of small doses of Viagra, 25 milligrams, one hour before the sexual act. Viagra does not prevent premature ejaculation but allows erection to last at least thirty minutes. This way the man may continue the sexual act until his partner has an orgasm. An important detail has to do with the woman's reaction if she realizes that her partner has ejaculated prematurely anyway. Open communication warning the woman about what might happen will help her accept it. Viagra may also be useful in the treatment of premature ejaculation following the techniques explained above.

Another method to prevent premature ejaculation is to suggest to young men that when the begin masturbating they should delay the moment of ejaculation and prolong the time period between stimulus and orgasm. The easiest way to do this is to stop as soon as a sensation of pleasure is felt, wait a few minutes and then resume masturbating. This may be repeated up to ten times before allowing ejaculation to occur. Basically it is the same conditioning mechanism for the treatment of premature ejaculation.

Delayed Ejaculation

Contrary to premature ejaculation, a man with delayed ejaculation takes some time to ejaculate. It is difficult to determine what is a normal period of time required for ejaculation and orgasm. This can only be decided with respect to the time the man needed before he started experiencing a delay.

It is not known how frequent this syndrome is. It is rare for the man experiencing it to complain or be uncomfortable, unless he cannot have an orgasm at all. I have observed this clinically in a very small number of patients. It is most likely to occur in patients over 50 or 60 who have had a prosthesis placed in the corpora cavernosa of the penis to treat sexual impotence.

Delayed ejaculation has also been observed in 50 to 60 year old patients who have had intracavernous shots of papaverine to help get an erection. I know only one patient whose delayed ejaculation could be considered a conditioning effect. This subject, whom I was seeing for different reasons, mentioned that ever since he started having sex, ejaculation would occur about 40 minutes after vaginal penetration. He was personally not bothered by this, but some of his sexual partners would complain of how long he needed to get an orgasm. During a second or third sexual act within two or three hours, ejaculation would take longer than on the first act.

When asked about how old he was when he started masturbating, he said he was eleven. He attended a Catholic boarding school where students had voluntary weekly confessions. One of his confessors told him that the "pleasure" of masturbation was a sinful act and that it was dangerous for the mental health of young men. This made a big impression and he became fearful of getting some mental illness since he masturbated once or twice a week. From the confessor's words he got the idea that it was the "pleasure" that came with ejaculation that was dangerous, not the manipulation of his penis. For a while he reduced ejaculation and orgasm to twice a month, but continued masturbating as frequently as before, except he would stop when he started to feel pleasure. Basically what he did amounted to one of the techniques used to treat premature ejaculation. This way he tried to prevent the "pernicious"effects of ejaculation that his confessor had warned him against.

In short, delayed ejaculation is basically related to a diminished sensibility of the nerve terminals on the epithelium that covers the penile area right behind the glans. When this sensibility decreases drastically or completely disappears, there is erectile dysfunction.

The treatment of delayed ejaculation, which does not bother most patients, consists in prolonging stimulation of the penis during foreplay. In cases where this is not sufficient and the female partner is uncomfortable with the prolonged action of the penis in her vagina, it is advisable to stop penetration and continue with manual or oral stimulation until the man begins to feel pleasure. Once this happens, there can be vaginal penetration again and the man can have an orgasm. These patients normally need more vigorous stimulation than others. If the woman doles not have strong enough vaginal muscles, she can try keeping her legs together once vaginal penetration has occurred.

Masturbation

Masturbation is the erotic satisfaction caused by the auto-stimulation of one's genitals. Some authors include any type of stimulation regardless of the final outcome. In other words, the sexual act of self-stimulation need not end in an orgasm to be considered masturbation. Since self-stimulation is a necessary part of this act, stimulation by a partner is not considered masturbation as it involves two people. Masturbation is a private act. Studies of animal sexuality show that several species of monkeys engage in self-stimulation. This has also been observed in dogs, elephants, and male dolphins in captivity. In spite of the apparent naturalness of masturbation from an evolutionary point of view, most human societies have considered it as deviant behavior in adults. Ancient Greeks and Romans did not discuss masturbation extensively. Hippocrates believed that excessive loss of semen caused deterioration of the spinal cord.

Although the Bible does not openly condemn masturbation, Judaism and traditional Christianity consider it a sin. The Catholic Church has not changed its traditional stance, and still considers masturbation an "unnatural act", since it serves no reproductive purpose. In part, masturbation owes its bad image to the Swiss physician S. Tissot, who claimed that in addition to being a sin, it was an illness that needed treatment. Ever since, masturbation has been blamed for mental weakness, blindness, brain atrophy, epilepsy, lethargy, premature senility, etc. Due to these unfounded ideas, parents consider it important to prohibit boys and girls to engage in any activity that in their view has a sexual content or expression. The truth is that masturbation must be considered a normal aspect of sexuality.

Many authors believe that self-stimulation starts with birth. They base this idea on the fact that newly born boys have erections, and one to three-year-old's show interest in manipulating their genitals. But it is important to know that baby boys may have erections at an early age without this being a sexual expression. Erections at this age are the result of a reflex of the spinal cord, which does not have the necessary inhibitions due to the lack of myelinization of the still immature nervous system. In addition, irritation of the genital area due to dampness or skin infections may produce erections and manipulation of genitals by children.

It is very difficult to detect a sexual activity just on the basis of observation and even less so by questioning children this young. What is unfortunate is that until 1940 medical authorities considered masturbation as a cause of illness or insanity. Up until then a number of devices were recommended to prevent the handling of one's genitals. In addition, special diets were prescribed that eliminated cheese, eggs, and asparagus for dinner, as these products were believed to increase the likelihood of nocturnal emissions. Other measures were basically torture applied to the genitals. In spite of all these efforts masturbation still exists.

Studies done in the last 30 years show a considerable change in people's attitudes towards masturbation. A 1974 study of sexual attitudes and behavior by Morton Hunt published in Playboy Magazine concludes that one out of six men and women between the ages of 18 and 34 consider masturbation objectionable. The same author found that among men and women over 45 only one third of them objected to masturbation. In another study done about the same time, Arafrat and Cotton found that most of the young men and women who had never masturbated had abstained because they did not feel the desire to do it. 32% of young men and 14% of young women thought that masturbation was wasteful of energy, immoral and shameful. Only a small fraction of this group gave religious reasons or a sense of guilt as reasons for not masturbating.

We must stress that masturbation is not a sin. It is a natural part of our sexual development. It is not lack of psychological maturity for an adult to masturbate, and it does not create habits that might interfere with the development of a healthy sexual life. On the contrary, masturbation may be beneficial. For instance, it provides a pleasurable sexual outlet for people without sexual partners. It may also be beneficial for those who have stronger sexual urges than their partners at a particular time, and in general it is a pleasant way to release tension. Although it is true that many people use masturbation as a source of pleasure, many young men masturbate mainly to deal with frequent and prolonged erections as well as the secretion of lubricating fluids on their underwear. This situation can be very embarrassing and annoying for those who experience it. The only way of alleviating a prolonged and painful erection is to masturbate.

There is no definite technique for self-stimulation. Each individual practices it according to their desires and their circumstances. According to the studies of Masters and Johnson, women generally use the same technique of self-stimulation, varying only in time, movements and style. The most common form of female masturbation is stimulation of the clitoris, the mons veneris, or the lips of the vagina, applying pressure, friction, and massage with their fingers. Only a small percentage of women masturbate with a finger penetrating the vagina. The variation in the form of self-stimulation results from information obtained through conversations with other women or from magazines and videos. This may include pressure on the thighs, contact of the genitals with a pillow, a warms water shower, vibrators, etc.

Most men masturbate by massaging the penis with a hand with long movements allowing friction of the prepuce on the glans, slowly at the beginning, and then accelerating as the sensation increases until they reach an orgasm. This stimulation is relatively short, generally not more than five minutes.

For various reasons, teenagers masturbate as fast as possible, mainly to avoid being caught in the act. If masturbation is practiced frequently with the purpose of obtaining an orgasm as fast as possible, the individual predisposes himself to ejaculate very soon after stimulation of the penis. Clinical observation has shown that most of the young men that suffer from premature ejaculation during intercourse have a history of rapid ejaculation during masturbation. Frequent masturbation under these conditions leads to the formatioon of a reflex that facilitates a rapid response to sexual stimulation.

The treatment of premature ejaculation is directed specifically to the elimination of this conditioned reflex so as to prolong the time between stimulation and ejaculation. The techniques to reach this goal are described in the section on premature ejaculation.

Stress Reduction

I have included a chapter on stress based on my conviction that marriage involves responsibilities and obligations and is not immune to problems and frustrations whose emotional effects may interfere with the harmony of interpersonal relations between the couple and with their children, and provoke conflicts and difficulties for the family's well-being.

Modern life, with its constant and rapid changes, requires adaptations and adjustments in all aspects and activities of our daily existence.

Before the women's liberation movement reached an advanced and deep stage, couples would get married according to certain tacit norms which are now questioned and in some cases not accepted by society.

Nowadays women must re-examine their own role and lifestyle within a framework where assumptions and expectations are in conflict. The problem of reeducation and readjustment for young and older women may be overwhelming. Men must also adapt to a new role that may involve greater responsibility towards family and home. They have been pressured by women's new modes of behavior, and this may represent a threat to their traditional role. Some of the changes that need to be faced within this liberation movement include changes in family structure, greater mobility that splits families into smaller groups or nuclei, care of children by unmarried women, care of children by divorced parents, conflicts involving job and home obligations for working women, etc. Everybody is affected by these changes.

On the other hand, there are tensions associated with most of our activities that we are all subjected to just because we are human beings, such as those resulting from our responsibilities, working conditions, economic competition, personal difficulties, family conflicts, illnesses, loss of family members, divorce, separation, children's school problems, marriage, pregnancy, imprisonment, sexual difficulties and others. These are problems that we must somehow overcome in order to avoid the toxic effects of acute or chronic stress on our health and to make our coexistence more tolerable.

There are basically three sources of stress:

The first one is the environment. We must put up with the weather, noise, interpersonal demands, crowds, time pressures, work-related responsibilities, threats to our safety and self-image.

The second source is physiological: childhood, adolescence, and menopause for men and women; aging, illness, and accidents; lack of exercise, poor diets, sleeping disorders. All of these factors affect our organism. Additionally, changes or threats to the environment also affect our bodies.

The third source is our thoughts. The brain interprets and translates complex environmental changes and determines when to sound the alarm. The way we perceive, interpret, and classify our present experience and its anticipated outcome may produce relaxation or stress. For instance, if we take our boss's unsociable look to signal that our work is unsatisfactory, we will experience stress. If, on the other hand, we take it to indicate fatigue or personal preoccupation, it will not threaten us. Stress results from the way we interpret a situation. We must ask ourselves what is really happening and why, and then determine how it affects our wellbeing, or how it threatens us and what we can do to face this threat. A depressed or stressed person often decides that the situation is dangerous and that it cannot be faced.

THE FIGHT OR FLIGHT RESPONSE

Humans react to situations of acute or chronic stress in a predictable fashion dictated by our neurophysiology. This reaction is known as the fight or flight response, and it is well known in animals and primitive men, for whom it could be a matter of life or death.

This instinctive response has not been lost in humans, but it has become a highly developed reaction that has allowed men to survive and reproduce themselves.

The fight or flight response with its bodily changes, like increased blood pressure, accelerated breathing rhythm, metabolism, and heart palpitations, is activated any time there is a situation that requires adaptation or adjustment of our behavior.

The modern foundation for the significance of stress as a psychological problem was established at the beginning of the 20th century by Walter B. Cannon, a Harvard physiologist. He was the first to show that the fight or flight response involved biochemical changes that prepare the individual to face a threat. Primitive man needed a rapid discharge of energy to fight or flee in the face of danger.

The first important researcher of stress was Hans Selye, who discovered exactly what happens in the human organism during the fight or flight response.

Selye defined the three classic stages of stress: alarm, adaptation, and exhaustion. His intuitive and methodological genius allowed him to uncover his well-known triad of adrenal hypertrophy, thymo-lymphatic atrophy, and gastro-intestinal ulcerations. Any problem, real or imaginary, causes the cerebral cortex to send an alarm signal to the hypothalamus, which is the center of reactions to stress. The hypothalamus, in turn, stimulates the neurovegetative nervous system to implement a series of changes in the organism. As a result there is an increase in heartbeats, blood volume and arterial pressure. The individual starts to sweat. Hands and feet get cold as a result of the blood being transported directly from the limbs and the digestive system to the large muscles. This helps the individual to fight or escape. The diaphragm and the anus contract, the pupils dilate to increase visual perception, and audition gets sharper.

While this is happening there are other reactions that may have a prolonged negative effect if they are not controlled. The suprarenal glands start secreting corticosteroids, adrenalin, and epinephrine, which inhibit digestion, reproduction, growth, and inflammation. In other words, some of these important reactions keep you healthy and strong under normal circumstances.

The same mechanisms that trigger the response to stress may also stop it. As soon as the individual considers the situation no longer dangerous, the brain stops sending emergency signals to the cerebral trunk. This, in turn, stops sending emergency signals to the neurovegetative system. The hormones and chemicals that put the organism in a state of alert are quickly metabolized.

A few minutes after the danger signals stop being sent to the organism, the fight or flight response decreases and the individual returns to his normal state.

Stress is a non-specific response of the organism to emotions and of the mind to any demand on the individual. The symptoms are manifested as a consequence of the lack or insufficiency of the adaptive mechanisms. The most prominent pathological effects are manifested as neurovegetative disorders. Any system of the organism may be damaged to a greater or lesser extent. Thus some people develop arterial hypertension, peptic ulcers, colitis, etc., as a consequence of stress.

On the other hand, not everybody is equally susceptible to the harmful effects of stress. People with a rigid character, tenacious, mentally inflexible, running from one appointment to the next, ambitious, incapable of giving everything its due time, are the most susceptible to suffering adverse consequences from stress.

On the face of frustrations and failure, human beings seek the most pleasant way of living, but they are never completely happy. Their behavior must adapt to the framework tolerated by their social, cultural, economic, and religious environment.

The response to stress, especially when it is chronic, is manifested in different ways. If the conflict is intense and the adaptive mechanisms are insufficient, tension is expressed in the form of psychopathological symptoms like anxiety, depression, hallucinations, and delirium, which can add up to neurosis or even psychosis. If the discharge is through the central nervous system, there may be hysterical manifestations, like motor paralysis, blindness, muscle spasms, etc.

The neurovegetative system is the one most affected by stress, with the effects we have described above.

The inhibition of the reproductive system may result in the interruption of menstruation and ovulation. In men it may result in sexual impotence and loss of libido. Stress may produce changes in the respiratory system, resulting in asthma, bronchitis, and other respiratory disorders. Loss of insulin during reaction to stress may contribute to the development of diabetes. Stress may suspend repair and renovation of tissues, leading to bone decalcification, osteoporosis, and susceptibility to fractures. Inhibition of the immunological system increases susceptibility to illnesses. In addition, chronic stress may contribute to the development of headaches, muscular tension, fatigue, and arthritis. There is evidence that chronic stress leads to the continuous discharge of norepinephrine, which may contribute to the development of an even greater depression.

The relation between chronic stress, illness and aging is a research area that has interested the scientific community. Experts in geriatrics are in the process of studying the characteristics of the illness and the appearance of degenerative disorders. The threat of infectious diseases like tuberculosis, typhoid fever, pneumonia, and poliomyelitis has been replaced by that of "modern plagues" such as cardiovascular disorders, cancer, arthritis, respiratory disorders (like asthma and emphysema), and a greater incidence of depression.

Normal aging is accompanied by a natural weakening of the functions of the organism. However, many of the disorders mentioned above that show up in people of middle and old age are sensitive to stress. Clinicians ask themselves how it is that stress accelerates the process of aging and what can be done to combat it. As mentioned above, our organism adapts to any change that we face.

Interpersonal relations, and marriage in particular, may contribute to stress. Even under the best circumstances, when there is a mutual harmonious relationship, there are many other factors that may interfere with the individual's wellbeing. This is an unavoidable part of our existence.

METHODS OF RELAXATION

The realization that chronic stress has harmful effects on people's mental and physical health has emphasized the need to find a procedure to counteract its undesirable effects on the human organism. The relaxation techniques that are used to this effect are aimed at reducing or controlling the brain's response to stress. The reaction to stress begins with the perception of change by the cerebral cortex, which then sends signals to the hypothalamus ordering a response through hormonal changes that will then activate the autonomous neurovegetative system.

Although we do not know how these relaxation techniques act on the complex system composed of the cerebral cortex, the hypothalamus, and the neurovegetative system, there is scientific proof of their effectiveness. An example of this are the studies by the physician Herbert Benson published in his book The Relaxation Response. The effect of the relaxation techniques is based on the biochemical and physiological changes observed in individuals who are highly trained in Yoga, Zen, and especially in Transcendental Meditation. These changes have been confirmed in the laboratory through experiments involving biofeedback. These experiments have shown that the mind, under special conditions, can modify certain bodily functions, such as arterial pressure or bodily temperature, among others.

Benson's studies have been done primarily on Transcendental Meditation and they have shown a decrease in oxygen consumption, metabolism, heartbeat, respiratory rhythm, and lactic acid in the blood (which is high during a state of anxiety), and an increase of the alpha waves in the electroencephalogram.

We must understand that all these changes, which are opposite to the fight or flight response, are in no way exclusive to Transcendental Meditation. These effects are the consequence of diminished activity of the autonomous neurovegetative system.

The relaxation method most widely accepted in Western culture is Transcendental Meditation. It is difficult for Western people to think of this method as "meditation", since it evokes a mystical and exotic Oriental concept or the practice of Christian monks who spent hours in their monastery cells contemplating God. Psychologically, it is considered an "altered state of conscience", an expression that has become very popular in the last few years, appearing in hundreds of publications. During this altered state of conscience, the individual is capable of experiencing a sensation of ecstasy, identification with his own self, wellbeing, unity with a supreme being, calm, serenity, or a combination or synthesis of these feelings.

It is an altered state of consciousness simply because we do not experience it frequently and it does not occur spontaneously; it must be induced on purpose and consciously. This state is in no way a mystical experience or a religious ritual. It is a sensation similar to the state of wellbeing that is felt after a period of physical exercise without reaching fatigue. It is believed to be related to the production of endorphins by the brain.

The mechanism of Transcendental Meditation by which the mind controls certain activities and bodily changes consists of muscle relaxation. It is a known fact that during the states of tension and anxiety the production of lactic acid in the blood increases, due to greater muscular activity. It has been shown that injecting lactic acid in the blood triggers anxiety attacks in humans. Controlling muscular activity by any relaxation method decreases the production of lactic acid. This way the autonomous vegetative system stops operating, which prevents the occurrence of all the biochemical and physiological changes that accompany the state of alarm.

There are various techniques of relaxation. We have mentioned Yoga, Zen, and Transcendental Meditation. To these we must add Autogenic Training, Progressive Relaxation, and Deep Hypnosis, among the better known. In general, all techniques of relaxation share some basic elements

We must keep in mind that even though all these techniques have certain basic elements in common, monks who practice them do so for prolonged periods of time, since these practices constitute an important part of their mystical lives. On the other hand, they are not exposed to the daily pressures that common people are exposed to. Consequently, common folks are somehow handicapped in obtaining the beneficial results of relaxation exercises. These exercises must be practiced constantly and regularly. It is important to have an intentional voluntary disposition, with the expectation of obtaining the effects of relaxation through a pleasant sensation associated with breathing exercises.

For beginners the main thing is to have a quiet place or environment that allows the elimination of internal stimuli and external distractions. A comfortable quiet room is ideal.

The second element is mental concentration on a word or phrase that is constantly repeated. This feature is one of the main practices that Buddhists and Hindus utilize to calm the mind. It is called a Mantra, literally "that which saves those who reflect", that is, a sacred word or phrase with spiritual significance and power that may be mentally or overtly repeated. This repetition is done in synchrony with breathing for greater effect.

The purpose is to concentrate one's attention on the pleasing sensation of the state of rest, preventing the interference of ideas, preoccupations, and feelings that may cause distraction from one's purpose of relaxation.

The third element is to adopt a passive attitude that allows the individual's mind to be a blank slate free of thoughts and distractions. This passive attitude is considered the most essential factor in the triggering or awakening of the relaxation response.

The fourth element is to adopt a comfortable position that can be maintained without change for at least 30 minutes. Sitting or semi-sitting on a bed is highly recommended. Some people suggest kneeling, sitting with one's legs crossed, etc. What matters is for the individual to stay awake, since the more comfortable the position, the greater the tendency to fall asleep.

Through the duration of the exercises the subject must keep his or her eyes closed, breathe slowly through the nose, keep the legs and arms extended or semi-flexed, not cross the legs, maintain the arms at the side of the body and not crossed over the chest or the abdomen, since both crossing the legs or putting one's hands over the body cause physical sensations that prevent the desired state of relaxation. A middle size pillow under the knees provides a resting position for those individual that experience lumbar discomfort. The position of the hands must be symmetrical, palms facing downward, keeping the arms separated and parallel to the body at the same distance.

The rationale for these positions is that they facilitate identical perception of tactile sensations and at the same time produce the same sensation of relaxation on both sides of the body.

Although any relaxation technique can lead to the same positive results, I will describe one that has been very well received by my patients. The technique is in no way esoteric and is based on the pleasant sensation of wellbeing produced by mental concentration and attention to the respiratory rhythm. Concentrating only on inhaling and exhaling may be difficult for some people, since there may be interference of other thoughts that distract them from the aim of their initial concentration.

To prevent this type of distraction we have designed a mechanism that can keep the mind concentrated on the action of breathing. It consists of the introduction of emotionally neutral words at the moment of inhaling and exhaling. The relaxation technique may thus be divided into the following phases:

FIRST PHASE

The subject adopts the most comfortable position, sitting on a couch, armchair or lying in bed. He or she then concentrates on breathing, with a slower rhythm than normal.

At the beginning of inhalation, the subject mentally counts 'one', and then exhales slowly. The cycle continues in this way until the subject reaches the count of twenty.

SECOND PHASE

The subject initiates another cycle of slow breaths, counting mentally at the beginning of inhalation. Now, when exhalation starts the subject repeats the following words: "I want my mind and my body completely relaxed". This cycle is repeated twenty times.

If the subject loses the count during the first or second phase, he or she must start over again and repeat until the sequence is correct. Similarly, if during the exercises there are episodes of yawning, the subject must start over from the beginning.

If yawning becomes more frequent and cannot be controlled, the subject must go on to the third phase. The persistence of yawning is indicative that sleep is being induced. If this is the case, the subject may do the exercise in the position in which he or she normally sleeps.

Alcohol and sedatives must be avoided before the exercises.

THIRD PHASE

In this phase the subject continues breathing slowly while concentrating on the respiratory rhythm without counting or uttering any words.

The purpose of proceeding in this form is to facilitate the subject's mental concentration only on the act of breathing and to avoid the interference of thoughts or words alien to the exercise.

The execution of these three phases takes about ten minutes. These relaxation exercises must be done two or three hours after meals, so as to avoid the neurovegetative effect of digestion. The exercises may be repeated two or three times if so desired, and any time at night. In cases of insomnia, these exercises may induce normal sleep. If this is not the case, the relaxation exercises may anyway produce a sensation of rest equivalent to that obtained under normal sleep. There is no time limit for the third phase. Most likely the subject will fall into a normal state of sleep.

After daily practice of these exercises for several weeks, the subject will notice the effect of a very pleasing mental and bodily relaxation. Once the subject is able to control his or her mental concentration on the act of breathing, he or she may stop being conscious of arms and legs and be aware only of the upper abdomen, the thorax, the neck, and the head. Heartbeats and pulsations on the temples and neck may become more intense for a moment, and then disappear. The feeling of wellbeing and relaxation, as well as the lack of awareness of arms and legs and the reduction of arterial pressure are the most noticeable signs that the individual is benefiting from the relaxation exercises we have described.

Summing up, this technique includes all the elements found in other relaxation techniques. It could be said that it shows the influence of hypnotic suggestion in the repetition of "I want my mind and my body completely relaxed". This does not detract from its value, since the individual knows what to expect from the exercise.

The optimal result of relaxation depends on the daily practice of the exercises. Their repetition will facilitate the response of relaxation. The sensation of wellbeing that is obtained is probably related to the production of endorphins by the brain.

This relaxation technique does not take a lot of time, since it can be completed in less than twenty minutes. There is no mystical mystery in this mechanism. The effect of the verbal significance of relaxation triggers the organic response of the sensation of wellbeing.

Although it is true that any technique to induce relaxation may help prevent or attenuate the symptoms of stress, it is important to remember that other measures related to the individual's health and attitude are necessary. The use of relaxation techniques is only one part of the program and one cannot expect them to be responsible for everything.

It is advisable to do some kind of physical exercise daily or at least four times a week, in thirty to sixty minute sessions. Walking, riding a stationary bicycle, or doing aerobics are good examples of moderate physical activity that is not exhausting and provides the sense of pleasant wellbeing.

An important factor is a balanced diet and maintaining an adequate weight. We must not forget that overweight may also be a consequence of stress, which makes people eat more than they need and consume food not appropriate to their diet.

Another important aspect to attain the maximal benefit from the relaxation response is to find the best solution to the situations and problems that trigger stress in the first place. If the subject is incapable to find a solution on his or her own, it may be necessary to consult a psychotherapist.

If the individual is methodical and persevering in the practice of the relaxation exercises, he or she will experience a notable effect of pleasure during and after engaging in them. The sensation of physical and mental wellbeing obtained will generate in him or her a positive attitude that will allow them to continue with the program outlined above on a daily basis.

PERSONAL EXPERIENCE

When we described the essential elements of the relaxation technique, we mentioned the need to have a place that provides a calm and comfortable environment to facilitate mental concentration and allow the individual to focus attention on the respiratory rhythm during the relaxation exercises. Although this is extremely important for beginners, it is less so for someone with experience. A subject in training must be able to attain a state of relaxation and wellbeing even if the place where he or she practices the exercises is not ideal. This way the relaxation exercises may be practiced in different locations and at different times. It is important that the subject evaluate his or her disposition and attitude before initiating the exercises.

Once the program has been started the individual must periodically examine himself or herself to see what positive changes have occurred. Certain aspects must be evaluated from time to time in order to have a reference point that will allow the individual to appreciate the impact of the relaxation response on his or her personality, and see if there has been a change of lifestyle.

CONCENTRATION AND ATTENTION

The ability to concentrate and focus attention on the respiratory rhythm and the pleasant sensation associated with breathing is essential in order to obtain a positive result from the relaxation response.

The subject will have no difficulty in judging if he or she is capable of attaining and maintaining mental concentration and attention on the exercise. The more favorable the individual's disposition, the lesser the risk of interference by ideas and thoughts with the exercise routine.

The development of this ability may be very beneficial for the subject, since in the future it will facilitate concentration and attention on any task or problem facing him or her. The individual will also find that his or her perception, attitude, understanding, and discernment will all improve as a consequence of a better disposition.

CALM, SERENITY, SELF-CONTROL, PEACEFULNESS

As a result of the relaxation response, the subject will progressively notice a significant change in mental and physical relaxation that will contribute positively in bringing about changes in personal attitude and lifestyle.

The individual will be pleased with this change, which will make him or her more patient and more receptive to new ideas that he or she was unaware of because they did not match his or her lifestyle. This improved tolerance and change of attitude will make possible a more adequate and satisfactory interpersonal relationship.

Calm and serenity will enable the individual to assume a positive attitude when facing doubts and fears, particularly those pertaining to physical problems and situations of anxiety. It is worth mentioning what some subjects say: "Now I see things more clearly. Before the relaxation exercises I had trouble finding solutions and solving certain problems. Now what happens is that generally at night after the exercises I find the solution without having been thinking of them. It is difficult to understand. The best way to explain this is as if at that moment my mind is illuminated."

The relaxation response, through physical and psychological changes, causes the individual to experience a sense of wellbeing and, consequently, of happiness. These changes make the individual more resistant to pain and less reliant on analgesics, several of which may be addictive. Similarly, in cases of arterial hypertension, it is possible to reduce the antihypertensive medicines, which have undesirable side effects and may cause sexual dysfunction.

An important aspect of the positive aspects of the relaxation response is its effect on insomnia. Some individuals with a history of insomnia report that if they cannot go to sleep after the relaxation exercises, continuing their practice during the night allows them to stay in one comfortable position for hours under deep mental and physical relaxation. In some cases, this may lead to a normal state of sleep, but in other cases, people who do not seem to sleep, are nevertheless totally relaxed in the morning.

The relaxation response, as explained above, has an obvious effect on control of anxiety and a beneficial effect on the prevention and treatment of the effects of stress.

About the Author

Dr. Jorge Weibel was born in Chile in 1922. He entered the School of Medicine of the Universidad de Concepción in 1940. In 1944 he continued his medical education at the Universidad de Chile, where he obtained his degree as a surgeon in 1947. For the next few years he worked as an Assistant in the Chairs of Medical Propedeutics, Physiology, Biochemistry, and Neurology at the Universidad de Concepción. In 1951 he was appointed Professor of Psychopathology, Psychiatry, and Neurology at the Schools of Social Work and Nursing of Concepción under the authority of the Universidad de Chile. With

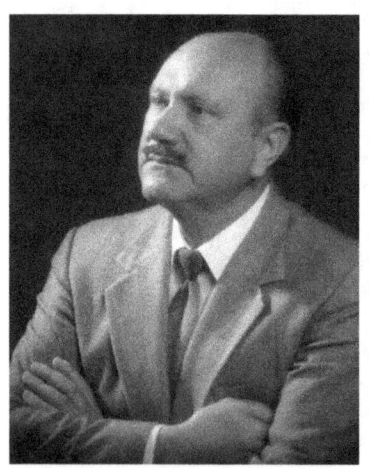

the creation of the Chairs of Neurology and Psychiatry at the Universidad de Concepción in the 1950's, he was appointed Assistant for both Chairs. In 1956 he travels to Houston, Texas to start a Residency in Neurology at the Baylor School of Medicine. He returns to Concepción in 1959. In 1961 he is hired as Assistant Professor of Neurology at the Baylor School of Medicine, a post he keeps until 1977.

In 1987 he is given recognition by the Medical Society of Concepción and Talcahuano on occasion of the society's 100th anniversary. In 1997 the Chilean government awards him the high distinction of the Bernardo O'Higgins Order in the rank of Officer, in recognition of his interest and dedication to the promotion and diffusion of Chilean cultural values, his humanitarian aid in the Santiago and Mexico earthquakes of 1985, and his outstanding professional and academic career during 50 years of professional activity. In 1997 he obtains official recognition by the Universidad de Chile on the occasion of 50 years of professional life and is appointed Visiting Professor of Neurology by the School of Medicine at the Universidad de Concepción.

He initiated his private practice in Concepción in 1959, and continued it in Houston. Since the beginning he had patients in his practice with erectile dysfunction and anorgasmia. The number of female patients was not very high since at the time there was widespread reluctance to discuss this type of problem. Later on this changed.

There were no classes on Human Sexuality in Schools of Medicine, so physicians lacked the most elemental knowledge to treat that kind of problem. The first statistical studies on male and female sexual behavior started in the 1940s. There was also an increased interest in psychotherapy and pharmacological treatment of sexual dysfunction, its psychological aspects, as well as the interpersonal factors that affect its origin and its solution. It became evident, as a conclusion of these studies, that interpersonal relations and harmonious coexistence of couples, as well as mutual sexual satisfaction were all very important. Furthermore, the effect on children since birth, and during their development and education, as well as after they become independent, is a very important factor in their future. We know that beginning at an early age humans imitate, learn and express their behavior.

These observations constitute the basis on which the content of this book is founded. I hope reading it will be helpful in developing stable interpersonal emotional relations with good understanding between parents and children.

References

Interpersonal Relationships

1. Buscaglia, Leo. Love. Ballantine Books, 1982.
2. Gray, John. Men, Women, and Relationships. Publishing, Inc., 1993.
3. Gray, John. Los hombres son de Martes. Las mujeres son de Venus. Editorial Atlantida, 1993.
4. Katz, Stand and Aimee Liu. False Love and Other Romantic Illusions. Ticknor and Fields, 1988.
5. Huston, T.L. and G. Levinger. Interpersonal Attraction and Relationships. Annual Review of Psychology 29:115-156, 1978.
6. Cecil Textbook of Medicine. 18th edition. W.B. Saunders Company, 1988.
7. El Manual Merk. Mosby/Doynua Libros. 9th Spanish edition, 1994.

Love

1. Casher, Lawrence. Is Marriage Necessary? Cited by Paul Gray, What is Love? Time, February 15, 1993.
2. Hatfield, Eliane. Love, Sex, and Intimacy: Their Psychology, Biology, and History. Cited by Paul Gray, What is Love? Time, February 15, 1993.
3. Lankowiak, William. Cited by Paul Gray. What is Love? Time, February 15, 1993.
4. Liebowitz, M.R. The Chemistry of Love. Little, Brown, 1983.

5. Fisher, Helen. Anatomy of Love: The Natural History of Monogamy, Adultery, and Divorce. Cited by Anastasia Toufexis. The Right Chemistry. Time, February 15, 1993.

6. Walsh, Anthony. The Science of Love and Its Effects on Mind and Body. Cited by Anastasia Toufexis. The Right Chemistry. Time, February 15, 1993.

7. Adams, Raymond D. and Victor, Maurice. Principles of Neurology. 4th edition. McGraw Hill, Inc. 1991.

8. Mitiguy, Judith, MS, RN. Neurologic Damage to the Anatomical Substrate for Sexual Functioning. Headlines, Jan/Feb. 1992.

9. Marañón, Gregorio. Obras Completas. Tomo X. Idearium. Madrid, Spain, 1977.

10. Buscaglia, Leo. Love. Ballantine Books, 1972.

11. Money, John. Cited by Paul Gray. What is Love? Time, February 15, 1993.

The Erotic Experience

1. Ferrer, Ferran. Cómo educar la sexualidad en la escuela. Ediciones Ceac. 1986.

Foreplay

1. Unseld-Baumanns, Christine. Erotic Partner Massage. Sterling Publishing Co. Inc. 1990.

2. Katchadourian, Herant. Human Sexuality. W.W. Norton and Co. Inc. 1972.

Anatomy of the Sexual Organs

1. Stoppard, Miriam. Woman's Body. Dorling Kindersley, 1994.

2. Clement, Carmine D. Gray's Anatomy. Williams and Wilkins, 1984.

3. Guyton, Arthur C. Textbook of Medical Physiology. 8th edition. W.B. Saunders Co., 1991.

4. Katchadourian, Herant. Human Sexuality. W.W. Norton and Co. Inc. 1972.

5. Masters, William H. and Virginia E. Johnson. Human Sexual Response. Little, Brown, and Co., 1966.

6. Masters, William H., Virginia E. Johnson, and Robert C. Kologny. Sexd and Human Loving. Little, Brown, and Co., 1988.

Sex Hormones

1. Guyton, Arthur C. Textbook of Medical Physiology. 8th edition. W.B. Saunders Co., 1991.

2. Wyn gaarden, James S., Lloyd H. Jr., and Bennet, J. Clande, Cecil. Textbook of Medicine. 19th edition. W.B. Saunders Co., 1992.

Physiology of Intercourse

1. Guyton, Arthur C. Textbook of Medical Physiology. 8th edition. W.B. Saunfkhjfders Co., 1991.

2. Smith, Donald R. General Urology. 11th edition. Lange Medical Publications. 1984

3. Heiman, Julia R. and Joseph Lopiccolo. Becoming Orgasmic. Prentice Hall Press. 1988.

4. Wyngaarden, James B., Joyd H. Smith, Jr., and J. Claude Bennet. Textbook of Medicine. 19th edition. W. B. Saunders Co., 1992.

5. Katchadourian, Herant. Human Sexuality. W.W. Norton and Co. Inc. 1972.

6. Grafenberg, Ernest. The Role of the Urethra in Female Orgasm. The International Journal of Sexology 3:145-148, 1950.

7. Gobberg, D.C. et al. The Grafenberg Spot and Female Ejaculation: A Review of Initial Hypothese. Journal of Sex and Marital Therapy 9:27-37, 1983.

Vaginal Penetration
Positions

1. Hooper, Anne. Pocket Kama Sutra. Carroll and Brown Limited. 1966.

2. Stoppard, Miriam. Woman's Body. Dorling Kindersley, 1994.

3. Katchadourian, Herant. Human Sexuality. W.W. Norton and Co. Inc. 1972.

Orgasm

1. Sexual Science: Bridging the Disciplines with the Master Clinicians. The Department of Continuing Education in Health Science, UCLA Extension, The School of Medicine, University of California, Los Angeles, 1987.

2. Heiman, Julia R. and Joseph Lopiccolo. Becoming Orgasmic. Prentice-Hall Press. 1988.

3. Carrera, M. Sex: The Facts, The Acts, and Your Feelings. Crown Publishers. 1981.

4. Friday, N. Forbidden Flowers: More Women Sexual Fantasies. Simon and Schuster. 1975.

5. Katchadourian, Herant. Human Sexuality. W.W.Norton and Co. Inc. 1972.

6. Kinsey, Albert C. et al Sexual Behavior in the Human Female. W.B. Saunders and Co., 1953.

7. Leiblum, S. et al. Vaginal Atrophy in the Postmenopausal Woman: The Importance of Sexual Activity and Hormones. Journal of the American Medical Association 249:2195-98, 1983.

8. Gebhard, P.H. Factors in Marital Orgasm. Journal of Social Issues 22(4):88-95. 1996.

9. Fisher, S. The Female Orgasm. New York: Basic Books, 1973.

Kegel's Vaginal Exercises

1. Kegel, Arnold. Sexual Functions of the Pubococeygeus Muscles. Western Journal of Surgery, Obstetrics, and Gynecology 60:521-524, 1952.

2. Heiman, Julia R. and Joseph Lopiccolo. Becoming Orgasmic. Prentice Hall Press. 1988.

3. Katchadourian, Herant. Human Sexuality. W.W. Norton and Co. Inc. 1972.

Oral Sex

1. Kinsey, Alfred C., W.B. Pomeroy, and C.E. Martin. Sexual Behavior in the Human Male. W.B.Saunders Co., 1948.

2. Kinsey, Alfred C. Sexual Behavior in the Human Female. W.B.Saunders Co., 1953.

3. Masters, William H. and Virginia E. Johnson. Human Sexual Response. Little, Brown and Co., 1966.

4. Masters, William H., Virginia E. Johnson, and Robert Kolodny. Sex and Human Loving. Little, Bown and Co., 1988.

5. Heiman, Julia R. and Joseph E. Lopiccolo. Becoming Orgasmic. Prentice Hall Press, 1988.

6. Calderone, May J. and Eric W. Johnson. Family Book about Sexuality. Harper and Row Publishers, 1989.

7. Katchadourian, Herant. Human Sexuality. W.W. Norton and Co. Inc., 1972.

8. Britton, Rosa de. La Costilla de Adán. Litografía e Imprenta Lil, S.A. Primera Edición, 1985.

Anal Sex

1. Masters, William H., Virginia E. Johnson, and Robert C. Kolodny. Sex and Human Loving. Little, Bown & Co. 1988

2. Heiman, Julia R. and Joseph Lopiccolo. Becoming Orgasmic. Prentice Hall Press, 1988.

3. Britton, Rosa de. La Costilla de Adán. Litografía e Imprenta Lil, S.A. Primera edición, 1985.

Premature Ejaculation

1. Sexual Science: Bridging the Disciplines with the Master Clinicians. The Department of Continuing Education in Health Science, UCLA Extension, the School of Medicine, University of California, Los Angeles, 1987.

2. Heiman, Julia R. and Joseph Lopiccolo. Becoming Orgasmic. Prentice Hall Press. 1988.

3. Masters, William H., Virginia E. Johnson, and Robert C. Kologny. Sex and Human Loving. Little, Brown, and Co. 1988.

Delayed Ejaculation

1. Masters, William H., Virginia E. Johnson, and Robert C. Kolodny. Sex and Human Loving. Little, Brown, and Co. 1988.

Masturbation

1. Herman, Julia R. and Joseph Lopiccolo. Becoming Orgasmic. Prentice Hall Press. 1988.

2. Masters, William H., Virginia E. Johnson, and Robert C. Kolodny. Sex and Human Loving. Little, Brown and Co., 1988.

3. Calderone, Mary S. and Eric W. Johnson. Family Book about Sexuality. Harper and Row. 1989.

4. Hunt, Morton. Sexual Behavior in the 1970s. Playboy Press. 1974.

5. Katchadourian, Herant. Human Sexuality. W.W. Norton and Co. Inc. 1972.

Stress Reduction

1. Davis, Martha, Elizabeth Robins, and Matthew McKay. The Relaxation and Stress Reduction Workbook. Future Health, Inc. Third Edition. 1991.

2. Benson, Herbert. The Relaxation Response. William Morrow and Company, Inc., 1975.

3. Selye, Hans M.D. The Stress of Life. Revised Edition. McGraw-Hill, 1976.

4. Mujica, Raúl M.D. Stress. Médico Interamericano, 34-36, 1986.